Removable Prosthodontics
at a Glance

This title is also available as an e-book.
For more details, please see www.wiley.com/buy/9781119510741

Removable Prosthodontics
at a Glance

Dr James Field

BSc(Hons) BDS PhD MFGDP RCSEng MFDS MPros
FDTFEd RCSEd CertClinEd MA(Ed) FAcadMEd PFHEA

Senior Specialist Clinical Teacher in Restorative
Dentistry & Consultant in Prosthodontics

National Teaching Fellow and Principal Fellow, HEA

Miss Claire Storey

BDS MSc MRes CertEd MFDS FDS RCSEng

Consultant and Specialist in Restorative Dentistry

WILEY Blackwell

This edition first published 2020
© 2020 John Wiley and Sons Ltd

The right of James Field and Claire Storey to be identified as the author(s) of this work has been asserted in accordance with law.

Registered Office(s)
John Wiley & Sons, Inc., 111 River Street, Hoboken, NJ 07030, USA
John Wiley & Sons Ltd, The Atrium, Southern Gate, Chichester, West Sussex, PO19 8SQ, UK

Editorial Office
9600 Garsington Road, Oxford, OX4 2DQ, UK

For details of our global editorial offices, customer services, and more information about Wiley products visit us at www.wiley.com.

Wiley also publishes its books in a variety of electronic formats and by print-on-demand. Some content that appears in standard print versions of this book may not be available in other formats.

Limit of Liability/Disclaimer of Warranty
The contents of this work are intended to further general scientific research, understanding, and discussion only and are not intended and should not be relied upon as recommending or promoting scientific method, diagnosis, or treatment by physicians for any particular patient. In view of ongoing research, equipment modifications, changes in governmental regulations, and the constant flow of information relating to the use of medicines, equipment, and devices, the reader is urged to review and evaluate the information provided in the package insert or instructions for each medicine, equipment, or device for, among other things, any changes in the instructions or indication of usage and for added warnings and precautions. While the publisher and authors have used their best efforts in preparing this work, they make no representations or warranties with respect to the accuracy or completeness of the contents of this work and specifically disclaim all warranties, including without limitation any implied warranties of merchantability or fitness for a particular purpose. No warranty may be created or extended by sales representatives, written sales materials or promotional statements for this work. The fact that an organization, website, or product is referred to in this work as a citation and/or potential source of further information does not mean that the publisher and authors endorse the information or services the organization, website, or product may provide or recommendations it may make. This work is sold with the understanding that the publisher is not engaged in rendering professional services. The advice and strategies contained herein may not be suitable for your situation. You should consult with a specialist where appropriate. Further, readers should be aware that websites listed in this work may have changed or disappeared between when this work was written and when it is read. Neither the publisher nor authors shall be liable for any loss of profit or any other commercial damages, including but not limited to special, incidental, consequential, or other damages.

Library of Congress Cataloging-in-Publication Data

Names: Field, James, 1979- author. | Storey, Claire, author.
Title: Removable prosthodontics at a glance / James Field, Claire Storey.
Description: Hoboken, NJ : Wiley-Blackwell, 2020. | Includes
   bibliographical references and index.
Identifiers: LCCN 2019056770 (print) | LCCN 2019056771 (ebook) | ISBN
   9781119510741 (paperback) | ISBN 9781119510710 (adobe pdf) | ISBN
   9781119510697 (epub)
Subjects: LCSH: Dentures. | Prosthodontics.
Classification: LCC RK656 .F495 2020 (print) | LCC RK656 (ebook) | DDC
   617.6/92—dc23
LC record available at https://lccn.loc.gov/2019056770
LC ebook record available at https://lccn.loc.gov/2019056771

Cover Design: Wiley
Cover Image: Courtesy of James Field

Printed and bound by CPI Group (UK) Ltd, Croydon, CR0 4YY

Set in Minion Pro 9.5/11.5 by Aptara Inc., New Delhi, India

10 9 8 7 6 5 4 3 2 1

Contents

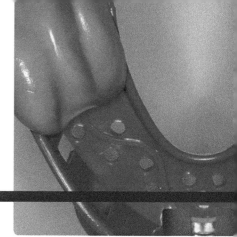

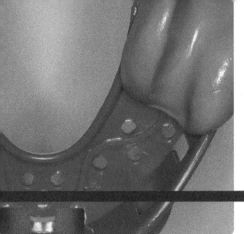

About the companion website

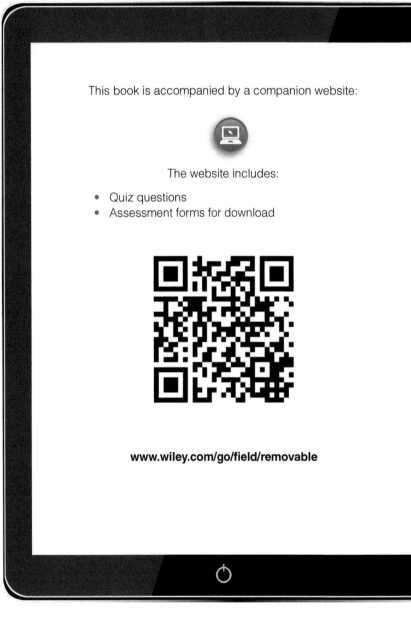

This book is accompanied by a companion website:

The website includes:

- Quiz questions
- Assessment forms for download

www.wiley.com/go/field/removable

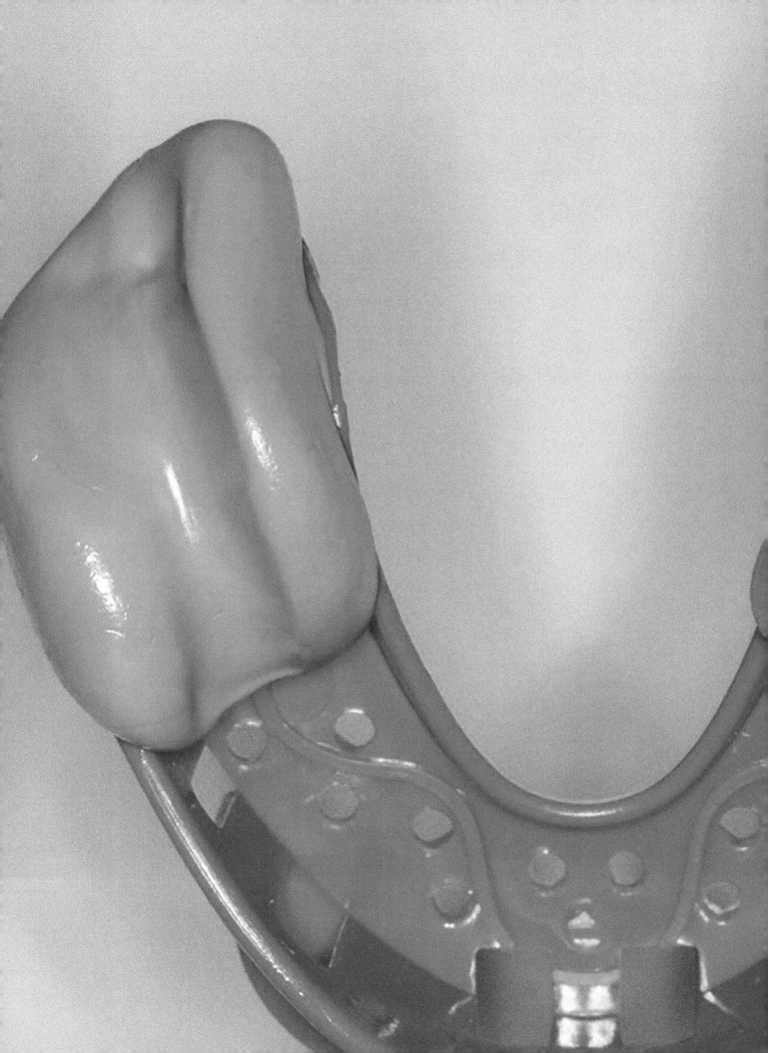

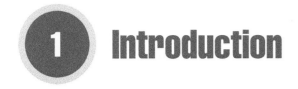

Introduction

Figure 1.1 Assessment processes

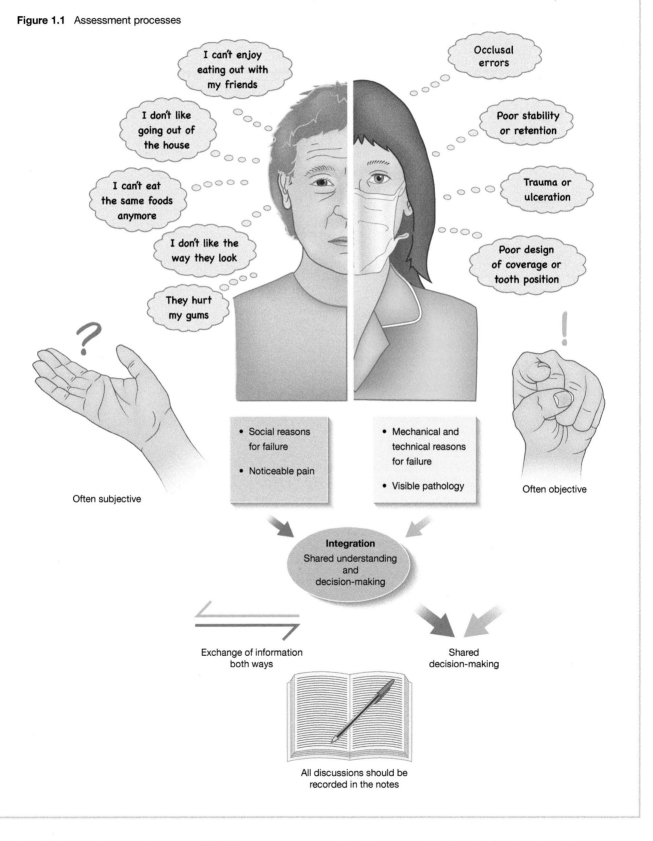

Removable Prosthodontics at a Glance, First Edition. James Field and Claire Storey. © 2020 James Field and Claire Storey. Published 2020 by John Wiley & Sons Ltd.
Companion Website: www.wiley.com/go/field/removable

Removable prosthodontics is often described as a 'black art' – the Marmite of dentistry; practitioners tend to either love it or hate it. Fortunately, we love it – and with some simple guidance, hopefully you will too. Like most operative interventions, success depends on:

- The skill of the dentist
- The technical difficulty of the case
- The patient's perceptions, ideas and expectations

Providing prostheses that are satisfactory to the patient is a challenge – and there are many reasons why patients can be dissatisfied with the finished result. Many relate to social aspects of patients' lives – how they are able to interact with others, particularly when eating and speaking. Common reasons include:

- Unacceptable aesthetics
- Inability to chew food properly
- Inability to enjoy the same foods as before
- Problems with speech
- Discomfort or persistent pain
- Disagreements over time and cost

Despite the diversity of complaints, there is often a common thread running through them all – lack of information exchange and an inappropriate level of patient expectation. We would therefore argue that the most important skill when making satisfactory removable prostheses is that of *communication*.

Communication and expectations

Effective communication takes *time*. As clinicians we often start looking for mechanical reasons to explain why patients might be having difficulties with their existing prostheses – excessive movement, trauma or ulceration, poor retention, or design of coverage. On that basis, we often agree to make a new prosthesis. In reality, patient tolerance relates to very much more than just mechanics and physical function. It is crucial that the treatment you provide is driven by *patient-perceived need*. This means that patients need to understand and buy into the clinical rationale, including risks and benefits, of the proposed treatment. Similarly, we need to understand the patient's rationale for wanting a prosthesis. Given enough time, it is highly likely that these requirements can be met.

Often, the process of making removable prostheses begins with a primary impression. Try and break that habit, and implement these simple steps first:

1 Set aside at least 5 minutes to talk to your patient
2 Sit in front of your patient – do not stand in front of your patient with a stock tray in your hand!
3 *Invite* your patient to explain why they would like you to make a denture – what are they hoping it will provide?

Crucially, your patient needs to feel that they can talk freely and comfortably about their tooth loss. This will not happen if they feel rushed, or feel that you are not actively *listening* to them.

This incredibly important part of the process is *investigative*. It should determine the choice of treatment that will follow. If the patient has an existing prosthesis, ensure that you ask what they think might change with a new one? What would they *like* to change?

It is at this early stage that you can begin to modify your patient's expectations if you feel that they are unrealistic. It is always better to begin this way, than back-tracking later and trying to reduce high expectations at the try-in or the fitting stages.

It is also a good opportunity to provide your honest thoughts on the likely outcome. We would caution against promising patients that their new prosthesis will be any better than the one that is being replaced, even if you can identify significant technical flaws. Instead, it is beneficial to ensure that you:

- Reiterate why you think the patient would like a new prosthesis
- Describe any technical features that you believe you can improve upon
- Estimate how many visits, including retries and review appointments, you expect may be needed
- Explain the fact that when the new prosthesis is fitted, even if it is technically better, it will still take a period of acclimatisation (up to 6 months, and longer in some cases) before the patient is able to function optimally
- Generate an understanding that during this time, the patient will need to adapt *slowly* to their new prosthesis, even if it appears to function comfortably – and this is particularly important in relation to complete denture patients

The clinical process

Communication aside, the process of making removable prostheses is more manageable than it may seem at first. There are often simple approaches that can yield excellent results, without expensive materials or equipment. In the main, technical success is about attention to detail and knowing which materials work best in your hands.

The aim of this at-a-glance guide is to provide advice on how to achieve optimal outcomes at each clinical stage of the process. Our opinions are based on decades of combined experience teaching at undergraduate and postgraduate level, and routinely treating a wide range of cases. We have provided recommended reading for each chapter in case you wish to read more about the technical stages, or to understand better the theory and evidence base that underpins the fabrication of removable prostheses.

Educationally, we use the term 'bricolage' (tinkering) when we are teaching our students about new materials in the clinics. If it has been a while since you have used some of the materials in this book, then get hold of some of them, and have a play!

2 The function of removable prostheses

Figure 2.1 The function of removable prostheses

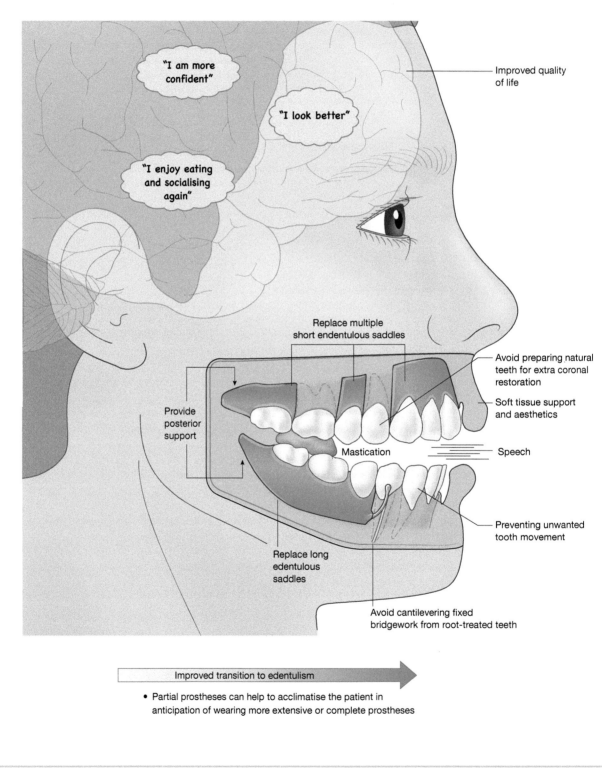

- Partial prostheses can help to acclimatise the patient in anticipation of wearing more extensive or complete prostheses

Function

It is often assumed that the function of a prosthesis relates only to 'mastication' – but there are many other functions that removable prostheses can serve. As clinicians, we are often good at recognising technical reasons why dentures should be constructed – but often the social aspects from the patient's perspective are overlooked.

Be mindful that the prosthesis must serve a function as perceived by the patient. If we are constructing a prosthesis that has a clear clinical rationale, but the reasons are less obvious to the patient, then we must spend time explaining how we intend the prosthesis to help. Unless the patient understands and believes the rationale for their construction, they are unlikely to wear them regularly.

That said, it is remarkable what patients *will* tolerate in order to achieve a desired outcome. For example, a patient might wear their prostheses whilst they are out of the house in order to facilitate a more normal social life – even if it is painful – but it is likely that they will take them out once they enter the house again – especially if they live alone. This is probably not dissimilar to us kicking off a pair of shoes that have been rubbing – but made us look good. Many patients living alone also take their dentures out in order to eat – so do not always think that the primary function of your lovingly constructed dentures is to help your patient to chew!

It is important to remember that replacement of all of the patient's missing teeth is often unnecessary. That said, it is still critically important that denture bases are extended into the full denture-bearing area in order to maximise stability and retention – and this will be discussed further in the following chapters.

Removable prostheses are indicated primarily for the following *clinical* reasons (Figure 2.1):
* Restoring masticatory function
* Restoring appearance
* Restoring speech
* Restoring soft tissue bulk and providing soft tissue support
* Acclimatisation during the transition to becoming edentulous

Removable prostheses are often indicated for the following *technical* reasons:
* Restoring long edentulous saddles
* Restoring multiple short edentulous saddles
* Providing posterior stability and improving occlusal load distribution
* Preventing undesirable tooth movements
* Rehabilitating to an increased vertical dimension
* Facilitating functional anterior guidance
* In order to prescribe diastemata between prosthetic teeth
* To avoid preparing abutment teeth for fixed prostheses
* To avoid cantilevering from root-treated teeth
* To aid planning and diagnosis, especially prior to implant placement

Finally, but by no means least, our patients may well request removable prostheses in order to:
* Improve aesthetics
* Restore social confidence
* Improve their eating experience

Restoring vs improving

Notice that most of the clinical rationale is based around *restoring* or *rehabilitating*, whilst patient requests often centre around *improving*. This important subtlety can easily be lost when negotiating informed consent. Correcting technical deficiencies and restoring clinical function does not necessarily result in a patient-perceived improvement. Again, moderating patient expectations is critical at each stage of treatment.

Quality of life

One of the most profound moments as an undergraduate was when Professor Janice Ellis (Newcastle) asked us whether we would rather lose a leg, and have a prosthetic replacement, or lose all of our teeth and wear a denture? At the time this seemed like a ridiculous comparison to make – but actually as clinicians we do become desensitised to seeing edentulous patients or partially dentate patients. The bottom line is whether we *really* sympathise with our patients or not. By working on a daily basis with edentulous patients who are struggling to cope, it is relatively easy to sympathise with the condition – even if we are unable to fully empathise. However, if we converse with denture-wearers less frequently, then there is a chance that we forget about what Professor Ellis termed the 'edentulous plight'. This reiterates why it is important that we take the time to *listen* to what our patients want, and that they feel comfortable enough to tell us.

Risks of removable prostheses

One of the most significantly overlooked aspects of denture provision is the potential negative impact on the hard and soft tissues. Primarily this relates more to the provision of partial prostheses – and patients should be made aware as part of the planning process (through informed consent) of the risks and benefits of receiving dentures. Do not assume that because your patient is already wearing dentures that there is no need to reiterate the potential risks.

Whilst the jury is probably out in terms of the impact on periodontal disease, there is clear evidence of an increased risk of plaque accumulation, gingivitis and root caries for patients wearing partial prostheses. Many well-conducted studies show that the key to minimising soft and hard tissue damage whilst wearing dentures is to maintain an optimal level of oral hygiene, and to attend regular review and maintenance appointments; this is very much a shared responsibility between clinician and patient. The patient must understand this, and the discussion should be well documented in the case notes.

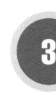

3 Stability and retention

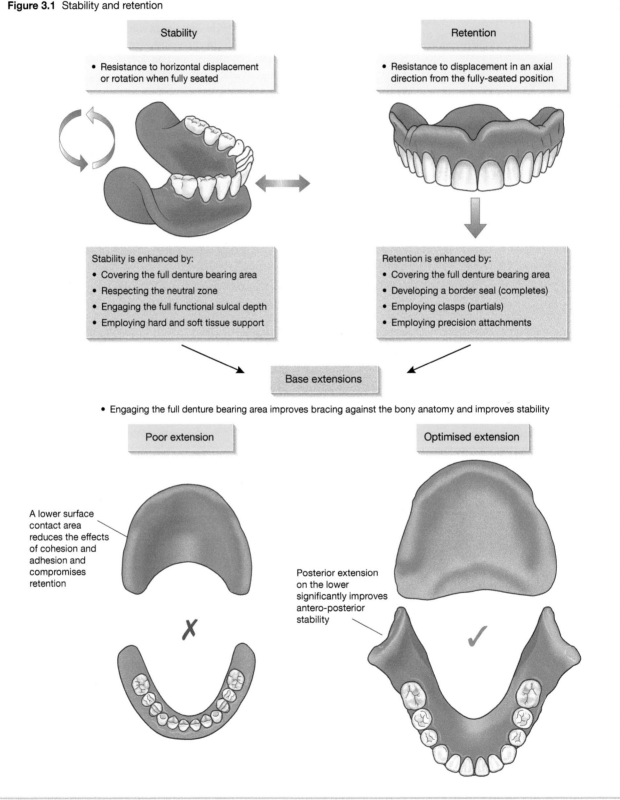

Figure 3.1 Stability and retention

Stability
- Resistance to horizontal displacement or rotation when fully seated

Retention
- Resistance to displacement in an axial direction from the fully-seated position

Stability is enhanced by:
- Covering the full denture bearing area
- Respecting the neutral zone
- Engaging the full functional sulcal depth
- Employing hard and soft tissue support

Retention is enhanced by:
- Covering the full denture bearing area
- Developing a border seal (completes)
- Employing clasps (partials)
- Employing precision attachments

Base extensions
- Engaging the full denture bearing area improves bracing against the bony anatomy and improves stability

Poor extension
A lower surface contact area reduces the effects of cohesion and adhesion and compromises retention

Optimised extension
Posterior extension on the lower significantly improves antero-posterior stability

Removable Prosthodontics at a Glance, First Edition. James Field and Claire Storey. © 2020 James Field and Claire Storey. Published 2020 by John Wiley & Sons Ltd.
Companion Website: www.wiley.com/go/field/removable

Stability and retention are fundamental principles for the construction of removable prostheses – consequently, problems with retention and stability often underpin the patient's perception of the prostheses.

Stability

This can be defined as the resistance to horizontal displacement or rotation – in complete dentures, or around large saddles, this is often determined by the underlying anatomy and ridge form; this is primarily assessed in terms of the cross-sectional profile of the ridge, and how much support the ridge is able to provide before it distorts or displaces.

From time to time you will notice ridges that present with fibrous aspects, which have a tendency to displace on palpation and loading. You may notice these presentations being referred to as flabby ridges, but this expression is not so well received with patients! Fibrous elements can affect the whole aspect of the ridge, or just the crestal tissues. The impact this has on denture stability will be determined by which anatomical features are affected and is discussed further in Chapter 17.

When considering shorter or bounded saddles, elements of stability will be derived from the way in which the denture base contacts the hard tissues (either acrylic or cobalt chrome) and engages undercuts. This is largely determined by the 'path of insertion' (POI) and is discussed further in Chapter 32. To a degree, the stability of the prosthesis is therefore dependent on how effectively the neighbouring teeth can support lateral loading. This is known as 'bracing'. If there is inadequate bony support for the abutment teeth then they will also move pathologically, and cause denture instability. This will cause further damage, possibly resulting in secondary occlusal trauma. These aspects will be discussed further, later in the book, in relation to partial denture planning.

Retention

This can be defined as the ability of the prosthesis to withstand removal in an axial direction – with complete dentures or areas over large saddles, this is often determined by the degree of coverage (employing cohesive and adhesive contact forces) and whether a border seal can be achieved. It is also important to consider the extensions of the prosthesis when assessing retention – whilst the prosthesis might be stable when fully seated, overextension may cause a lack of retention in function, as the functional sulcus shortens and displaces the denture base. When considering partial dentures and implant-supported overdentures (ISOD), retention becomes a much more active concept, through the use of direct clasps and retentive abutments. ISODs are considered further in Chapter 41.

Stability vs retention

I am often asked whether a denture can be stable yet unretentive – and vice versa. The simple answer is yes – to both. The technical challenge comes in ensuring that the prosthesis demonstrates both stability *and* retention. The key here is that the prosthesis covers the full denture bearing area – and accommodates functional movements within the periphery – the functional sulcus.

We will revisit the full anatomy of the maxillary and mandibular denture bearing areas (DBA) later – but some important anatomical and functional considerations for stability include:

- The form of the edentulous ridge and palate
- The degree of support offered by the ridges
- The position of the polished surfaces in relation to the neutral zone (Chapter 24)
- The degree to which the maxillary tuberosities are fully captured
- The degree to which the disto-lingual anatomy is captured

Patients tend to learn how to improve the stability of dentures by improving muscle tone, tongue control and chewing habits. Whilst edentulous patients often have a habit of improving retention by holding dentures up with the posterior dorsum of the tongue, this appears to be a very patient-specific skill.

Important anatomical aspects for retention include:

- Full coverage of the DBA
- Developing an adequate border seal
  - Fully capture the maxillary tuberosities
  - Fully capture the lingual anatomy
  - Accounting for the insertion of buccinators into the retromolar pad
- Ensuring that the denture is adequately extended, but not overextended, in function

Whilst the DBA and its extensions are very important, the position of the teeth is also critical, particularly in relation to the labio-lingual position of incisors on a lower complete denture. The concept of the neutral zone is very important and this will also be discussed later in Chapter 24. As well as the neutral zone, and impressions to record it, there are other prosthodontic techniques that can be employed to overcome challenges with fibrous ridges – such as:

- The RPI design principle
- The Altered Cast technique
- Various mucostatic or mucocompressive impression techniques

These will be discussed further later in the book.

The gag reflex

This is discussed in more detail in Chapter 46 – however, it is worth mentioning at this early stage that the vast majority of patients presenting with a gag reflex are anticipating movement or loss of retention of their prosthesis. It may be that their current prosthesis *is* stable and retentive – however, most often I find that this is not the case. It is important to take the time to explain to patients that the best outcome is achieved if a stable and retentive denture is created first, which can then be used as a predictable tool for overcoming a gag reflex. Even in patients where counselling is required in order to overcome psychosocial triggers, a well-fitting prosthesis is necessarily the starting point.

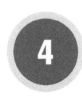

Patient assessment for complete dentures

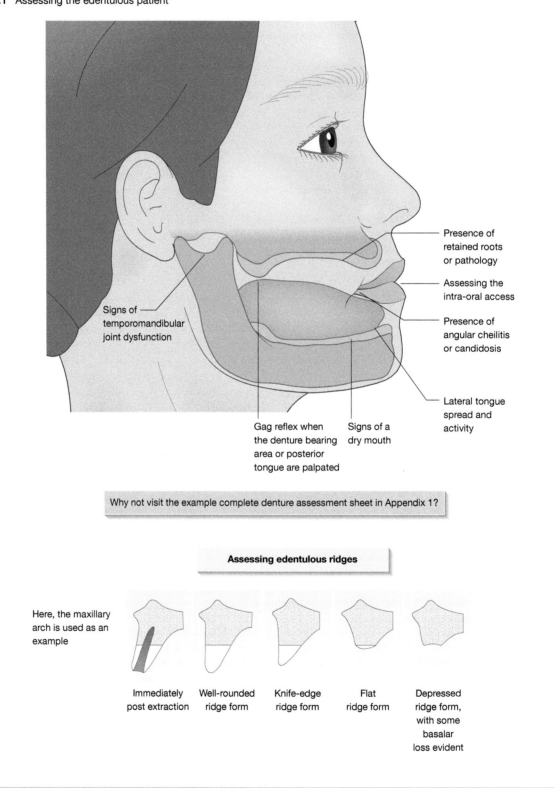

Figure 4.1 Assessing the edentulous patient

Signs of temporomandibular joint dysfunction

Presence of retained roots or pathology

Assessing the intra-oral access

Presence of angular cheilitis or candidosis

Lateral tongue spread and activity

Gag reflex when the denture bearing area or posterior tongue are palpated

Signs of a dry mouth

Why not visit the example complete denture assessment sheet in Appendix 1?

Assessing edentulous ridges

Here, the maxillary arch is used as an example

Immediately post extraction

Well-rounded ridge form

Knife-edge ridge form

Flat ridge form

Depressed ridge form, with some basalar loss evident

Removable Prosthodontics at a Glance, First Edition. James Field and Claire Storey. © 2020 James Field and Claire Storey. Published 2020 by John Wiley & Sons Ltd.
Companion Website: www.wiley.com/go/field/removable

Arguably one of the most important elements of your patient assessment, is about taking the time to understand what the patient wants and why. It is also about making a judgement about how likely you are to succeed with your endeavours – there are a number of risk factors that can alter your chances of success and these should be discussed and recorded before the active elements of treatment begin. The majority of these factors are outlined below, largely as bullet point questions, but please do visit the recommended reading section for details of other academic texts which explore some of these concepts in further detail. Please also see the sample Complete Denture Assessment Proforma in Appendix 1.

The patient and the rationale for treatment

- Why does the patient want new or improved dentures?
- Is there any difficulty chewing or speaking?
- Do the dentures cause pain or nausea?
- Do the dentures cause gagging, and if so, is it immediate?
- Are the dentures of a satisfactory appearance?
- Have any of these problems got worse recently?

Prosthodontic history

- What type of denture is the patient currently wearing?
- How old is the prosthesis and where was it/they made?
- For how many years has the patient been edentulous?
- How many prostheses has the patient received before?
- Is the patient willing to attend for the necessary appointments, including review appointments?

Clinical examination

Before considering removable complete prostheses, it is important to carry out a full and comprehensive extra- and intraoral assessment. The following aspects can then be considered (Figure 4.1).

- *Intraoral access* – Can the full denture-bearing anatomy be palpated easily, and can the existing prostheses be easily inserted and removed from the mouth?
- *Tongue* – Does this occupy a normal space, or does it exhibit lateral spread? Is there a habit of using the tongue to retain the upper denture posteriorly?
- *Gag reflex* – Can the full denture-bearing area be palpated without eliciting a gag reflex? If not, where are the trigger zones? These are most often the dorsum of the tongue, or the posterior palate.
- *Ulceration* – Are there any existing signs of ulceration, and do they correspond to the extensions of a prosthesis?
- *Temporomandibular disorder (TMD)* – Are there currently any signs of muscle pain or temporomandibular joint (TMJ) derangement?
- *Candidosis and angular cheilitis* – How old are the prostheses and what is the patient's current hygiene regime? Does the patient seem to be over-closed? Is there a high carbohydrate intake throughout the day, nutritional deficiency or a dry mouth?
- *Dry mouth* – Does the patient complain of a dry mouth? Is this medication-induced? You can grade a dry mouth using the Challacombe scale (see recommended reading).

- *Tori or significantly undercut ridges* – If present will these interfere with the denture extensions or path of insertion?
- *Retained roots* – Could these be retained as overdenture abutments?
- *Any suspicious lesions*, particularly for at-risk patients, that should be investigated or monitored alongside treatment?

Ridge assessment

Manual palpation is very important in order to assess the ridges adequately. This includes the ridge form (Figure 4.1) (well-formed, atrophic, rounded, flat, knife-edge, fibrous, undercut) and the proximity of the frenal attachments to the crest of the ridges.

Assessment of existing prostheses

The *stability* (resistance to horizontal or rotational displacement when fully seated) and *retention* (resistance to vertical displacement) of each prosthesis should be assessed in turn. It is easier to do this individually rather than having both prostheses in at the same time. The upper should be seated from in front of the patient, and whilst holding the molar units, should be rotated in a horizontal plane. It can then be displaced vertically, ensuring that the patient is not holding the denture in place with their tongue, to assess retention. The lower should also be seated from in front of the patient, ideally with the patient in a seated position. Stability can be assessed as above, but also in an antero-posterior direction by pinching the lower incisors between thumb and forefinger and moving the denture lingually and labially.

The denture *extensions* should then be considered – labial, buccal and posterior aspects – but also coverage of the tuberosities on the upper and disto-lingual extension on the lower. The anatomy of the denture-bearing area is considered in Chapter 10. It is important to assess the extensions systematically to look for under- or overextension. Direct vision is possible for the lower but it can be more challenging on the upper. Retracting the sulcus with your index finger parallel to the arch means that as you seat the denture, you can feel whether the sulcus is 'pulled in' towards the prosthesis. If this is the case, the denture is overextended in this area. It is also possible to take a wash impression in silicone or alginate to assess the denture extensions at this stage.

In terms of *aesthetics* – lip support, incisal plane and buccal space should be noted. These are considered further in Chapter 20.

Finally, in relation to the *occlusion*, it is important to note whether the intercuspal position is stable and whether there are any heavy contacts. Is the intercuspal position coincident with the retruded arc of closure – and if not, what are the characteristics of the slide? Finally, assessment should be made of the freeway space between the dentures – although at this stage an estimate can be made by listening to the 'speaking space' available – sibilant sounds will sound sharp and whistle-like if the freeway space is restricted, and hollow or absent, if it is excessive.

At this point, a diagnosis can be made with a suitable prognosis (and justification), and your patient's expectations can be discussed in an informed way. A treatment plan can be devised relating to the fitting surface, the occlusal surface and aesthetics (polished surfaces).

5 Edentulous ridge presentations

Figure 5.1 Edentulous ridge presentations

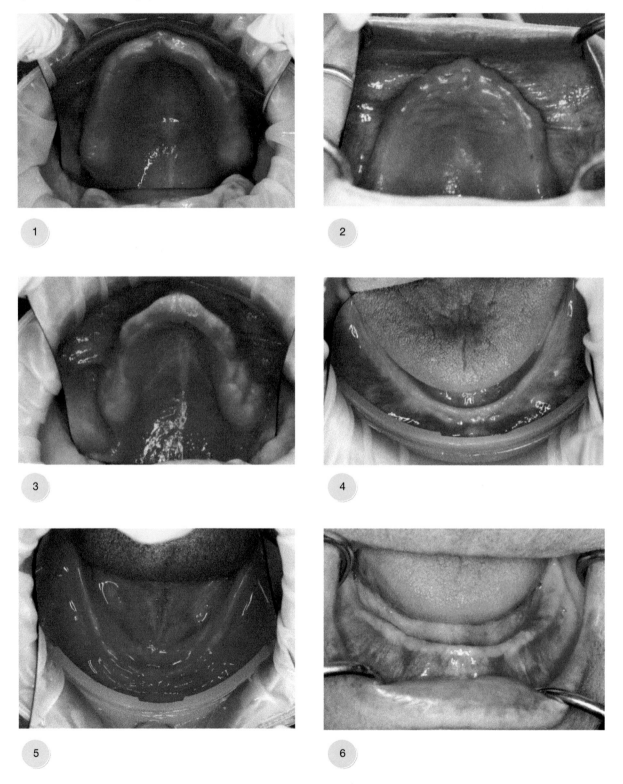

Removable Prosthodontics at a Glance, First Edition. James Field and Claire Storey. © 2020 James Field and Claire Storey. Published 2020 by John Wiley & Sons Ltd.
Companion Website: www.wiley.com/go/field/removable

The photographs opposite show a range of edentulous ridge presentations. Whilst the range shown is by no means exhaustive, each photograph presents a number of interesting points for consideration when planning a removable prosthesis.

Upper edentulous ridges

Photograph 1

Intraoral access here is good and the full denture-bearing area (DBA) can be palpated without any pain or gagging. The mucosa looks moist and there are no signs clinically of a dry mouth. The ridge is well formed with high and rounded ridges – and this would be classified as Class III (Cawood and Howell). A retained root has recently been extracted from the UL5 and this presents as a crestal defect. The prominent incisive papilla is erythematous and this is a sign that it may need a degree of relief in order to prevent recurrent trauma. There is a slight buccal defect to the ridge on the left-hand side and the muscle attachment here inserts into the base of the sulcus. Paradoxically it can be easier to account for high muscle insertions than lower ones – and so this area would receive particular attention during the working impression. It is possible to see the posterior extent of the existing denture, which is short of the fovea palatini by at least 10 mm. It is also possible to see the limited degree to which the denture base wraps around the tuberosity on the right-hand side – and this can be improved during the working impression with a border moulding material to ensure that its full anatomy is captured.

Photograph 2

Intraoral access here is slightly restricted. The full DBA can be palpated without pain or gagging. The mucosa looks shiny and dry, and clinically there are signs of a dry mouth; the mirrors stick to the mucosa, and food debris accumulates at the denture borders. It may be necessary for the patient to consider a saliva substitute in order to promote effective adhesion and cohesion, and a border seal. The ridge is well defined and rounded (Class III), but the sulcal depth reduces significantly towards the posterior aspects. The palate is relatively shallow and broad – shallow ridges and a shallow palate mean that the denture may have a compromised stability. The muscle attachments insert onto the crest of the ridge – this is the other extreme of how attachments may present. The challenge here is ensuring they are accommodated for, without compromising the border seal. The labial portion of the anterior ridge presents with a significant undercut and it is worth considering at the assessment stage whether a defined path of insertion is possible, or whether the permanent base should be modified with permanent soft liner to allow the ridge to be atraumatically engaged.

Photograph 3

Intraoral access here is excellent. Palpation of the DBA in the palate beyond the posterior border of the existing prosthesis results in a gag reflex. There is no pain on palpation. The ridge is well formed (Class III) but lacks some definition in the premolar regions, where it presents with a knife edge (Class IV). Once again, muscle attachments are situated near the base of the sulcus, so attention to detail during the working impression will be important. It is possible to see the posterior extent of the existing denture, which is short by at least 15 mm. It is also possible to see the limited degree to which the denture base wraps around the tuberosities. Both of these features will significantly compromise the stability and retention, and perpetuate the gag reflex. A thin band of tissue exists along the crest of the ridge from incisor to premolar on the patient's right-hand side, and this should be accounted for in the working impression; in order to avoid the denture 'nipping' the tissues, the impression should be taken in zinc oxide eugenol, and the borders of the thin tissue ridge should be filleted away with a scalpel. Once again, the labial portion of the anterior ridge presents with a significant undercut and it is worth considering at the assessment stage whether a defined path of insertion is possible, or whether the permanent base should be modified with permanent soft liner to allow the ridge to be atraumatically engaged.

Lower edentulous ridges

Photograph 4

The full DBA can be palpated without any pain, although contact with the posterior lateral borders of the tongue elicits a gag reflex. The ridge is atrophic with a knife edge presentation (Class IV). A thin fibrous band of tissue runs along the entire crest of the ridge – and this should be accounted for in the working impression; in order to avoid the denture 'nipping' the tissues, the impression should be taken in zinc oxide eugenol, and the borders of the thin tissue ridge should be filleted away with a scalpel. Muscle attachments are low and there is only a moderate sulcal depth anteriorly when the lip is retracted. The tray will need to be carefully adjusted here to ensure it is not overextended.

Photograph 5

The full DBA can be palpated here without eliciting pain or a gag reflex. The tissues are fibrous anteriorly, and it is possible to see the folds of tissue in the photograph. The ridge is atrophic (Class V) but presents with an identifiable fibrous crest. This is thicker than in photograph 4, and so is unlikely to fold over when the denture is seated. No special interventions are required in that regard. There is little identifiable sulcus anteriorly and so the tray will need to be carefully adjusted here – and it may even be the case that a purposefully mucostatic or mucocompressive impression (depending on the assessment) is taken to account for the anterior fibrous tissue. Ulceration is visible in the buccal and labial sulci, and it is important to ensure that this is resolved prior to working impressions.

Photograph 6

The full DBA can be palpated without pain or gagging. The ridge is firm, well formed and generally rounded at the crest – although there are undercut aspects around the buccal aspect. This would be graded as Class IV. Muscle attachments are relatively low and there appears to be a reasonable depth to the labial sulcus. Avoid thinking that these cases are straightforward to treat – it is sometimes the case with well-formed ridges that they pose problems in terms of ridge pain after fitting of the dentures.

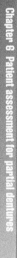

6 Patient assessment for partial dentures

Figure 6.1 Patient assessment for partial dentures

Assessment process

Patient history

Primary impressions

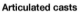

- Accurate, well extended
- Material supported by the tray
- Full sulcal recording
- Free from air blows, drags or tears

Articulated casts

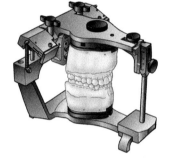

- Accurate articulation either in intercuspal position or at an increased occlusal vertical dimension

- For notes on accurate preliminary registration see chapters 19 and 29

Periodontal assessment

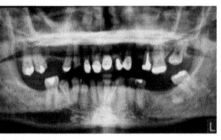

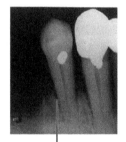

Basic periodontal examination (BPE) or 6 point pocket chart + mobility scores

Radiographic assessment of:
- Bony support for abutment teeth
- Root angulation of abutment teeth
- Pathology around abutment teeth

- Look out for crestal funnelling, indicative of occlusive trauma

Preliminary restorative work

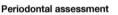

Consider:
- Additions to worn teeth
- Provision or replacement of extra coronal restoration
- Extractions of roots

Preliminary designs

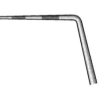

Marking teeth that are unable to support axial loads, can help you to design the partial denture more efficiently

Removable Prosthodontics at a Glance, First Edition. James Field and Claire Storey. © 2020 James Field and Claire Storey. Published 2020 by John Wiley & Sons Ltd.
Companion Website: www.wiley.com/go/field/removable

An assessment for a partial prosthesis begins in much the same way as for a complete denture – why does the patient want the treatment, and what are the risk factors that can alter your chances of success? The main obvious difference, however, is the presence of standing natural teeth. The health and prognosis for these teeth must be adequately assessed in order to plan the treatment effectively for removable partial prostheses – and whilst the method of partial denture design will be covered later, the necessary clinical information and indices will be mentioned here as part of the initial assessment stage.

The patient and the rationale for treatment

• Why does the patient want new or improved dentures?
• Do the current dentures cause pain?
• Is there any difficulty chewing or speaking?
• Are the dentures of a satisfactory appearance?

Prosthodontic history

• What type of denture is the patient currently wearing?
• How old is the prosthesis and where was it/they made?
• For how many years has the patient been wearing partial dentures?
• How many prostheses has the patient received before?
• Is the patient willing to attend for the necessary appointments, including review appointments?

Clinical examination

Before considering removable partial prostheses, it is important to carry out a full and comprehensive extra- and intraoral assessment. The following aspects can then be considered.
• *Intraoral access* – Can the denture-bearing anatomy be palpated easily, and can any existing prostheses be easily inserted and removed from the mouth?
• *Plaque control* – Wearing removable partial dentures in the presence of poor plaque control poses a significant risk to the dentition, for the progression of root caries and soft tissue disease. If the basic periodontal examination (BPE) codes are anything but 0, you should be carrying out at least a plaque score and providing tailored oral hygiene instruction.
• *Tooth mobility and periodontal pocket depths* – Whether teeth are pathologically mobile or present with deep bleeding pockets is often overlooked during a partial denture assessment. It is often assumed that the expected future loss of teeth warrants an acrylic partial denture – in reality, it is important to determine which teeth might be capable of helping to support a removable partial denture down their long axis, and use them accordingly. Teeth may also present with mobility because of occlusal trauma, especially if there is a lack of posterior support. This is unlikely to improve without the provision of a removable prosthesis to replace posterior units.
• *Gag reflex* – Can the denture-bearing area and connector sites be palpated without eliciting a gag reflex? If not, where are the trigger zones? These are most often the dorsum of the tongue, or the posterior palate.
• *Ulceration* – Are there any existing signs of ulceration, and do they correspond to the extensions of a prosthesis?

• *Temporomandibular disorder* – Are there currently any signs of muscle pain or temporomandibular joint derangement?
• *Dry mouth* – Does the patient complain of a dry mouth? Is this medication-induced? A dry mouth will significantly increase the risk of root caries and gingivitis when wearing a partial denture.
• *Retained roots* – Could these be retained as overdenture abutments and what is the space between root surface and opposing tooth? Do not forget that healthy retained roots will prevent alveolar resorption, improve proprioception and chewing ability. Further, there is a large psychological benefit to retaining natural teeth and tooth roots.
• *Worn or compromised teeth* – Could worn teeth be restored directly or indirectly prior to the provision of removable prostheses? Could the removable prosthesis overlay the worn teeth to restore their form and function? Can an extra coronal restoration be placed with elements that will facilitate partial denture stability and retention, such as milled shoulders, rest seats and guide planes. These are questions that are often overlooked when planning removable partial prostheses and will be discussed further later in the book.

Ridge assessment

Ridge form may be less critical with removable partial dentures, particularly if there are bounded saddles – but atrophic ridges and thin fibrous bands of tissues should still be noted, because these can cause problems, especially with free-end saddle presentations.

Partial denture classification

In relation to ridge and saddle configuration, it is important to be able to communicate the type of partial denture effectively to colleagues and the wider dental team. Chapter 28 describes the Kennedy partial denture classification system, which is probably the most ubiquitous. It is also very important to decide whether you will maintain the natural tooth contacts in the current intercuspal position, or whether you will be changing (or reorganising) the occlusion. It will not be possible to plan or design a partial denture effectively without deciding this first. This is covered further in Chapter 23.

Assessment of existing prostheses

Partial dentures should be assessed in the same way as for complete dentures in relation to retention and stability. It is, however, also important to appraise the connector design, and the path of insertion, even if the dentures are made totally in acrylic. Material choice and connectors are discussed later in Chapters 28 and 31.

Radiographic assessment

As well as a thorough periodontal and restorative assessment, it is important to assess potential abutment teeth radiographically for any potential periapical pathology and to assess the bony support available. It is also important to assess the angulation of the long axis of the tooth. Non-axially loading a tooth can exacerbate occlusal trauma and bony loss.

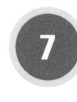 **7** # Factors complicating success

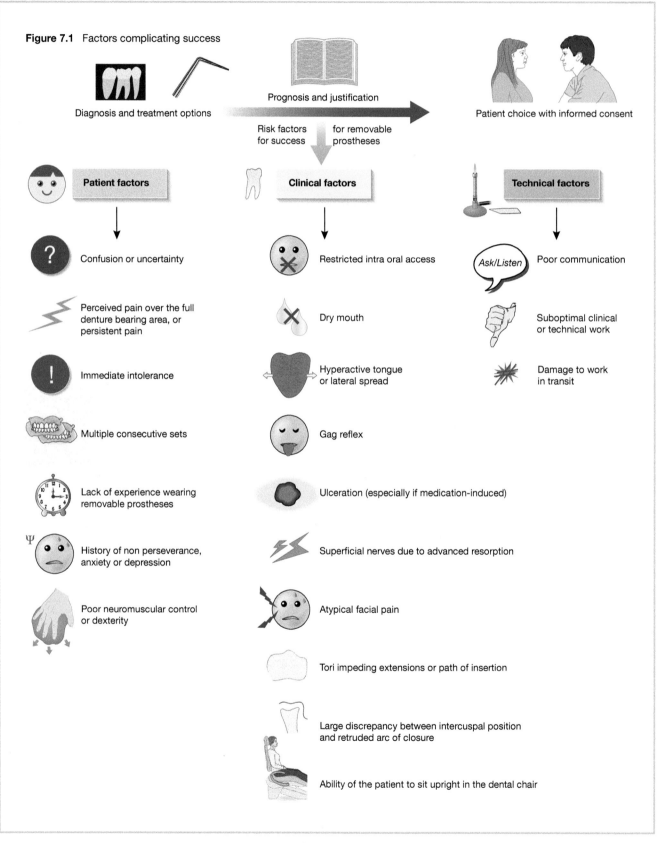

Figure 7.1 Factors complicating success

Diagnosis and treatment options

Prognosis and justification

Patient choice with informed consent

Risk factors for success for removable prostheses

Patient factors

Confusion or uncertainty

Perceived pain over the full denture bearing area, or persistent pain

Immediate intolerance

Multiple consecutive sets

Lack of experience wearing removable prostheses

History of non perseverance, anxiety or depression

Poor neuromuscular control or dexterity

Clinical factors

Restricted intra oral access

Dry mouth

Hyperactive tongue or lateral spread

Gag reflex

Ulceration (especially if medication-induced)

Superficial nerves due to advanced resorption

Atypical facial pain

Tori impeding extensions or path of insertion

Large discrepancy between intercuspal position and retruded arc of closure

Ability of the patient to sit upright in the dental chair

Technical factors

Ask/Listen — Poor communication

Suboptimal clinical or technical work

Damage to work in transit

Prognosis and justification

Each diagnosis and treatment plan should be qualified with a *prognosis* – an indication of the likely outcome of the condition, or the proposed treatment. Without this information, the patient is unable to make an informed choice about which treatment modality to pursue – and so it is important to remember to discuss this and record the discussions within the patient notes. Just as important as the prognosis is the *justification* for how this decision is reached. A comprehensive and thoroughly recorded assessment will facilitate this process. The factors below are considered to be risk factors when constructing removable prostheses (Figure 7.2).

Risk factors

Patient factors

• *Patient confusion or uncertainty* – If patients are unsure about why they are receiving a prosthesis, or they feel that there is little need, then they are less likely to wear the finished product. You must be clear about what your treatment aims are, and this should be checked and reinforced at each patient appointment.

• *Pain over the full denture-bearing area (DBA)* – An ache or a burning sensation over the entire DBA (on either arch) can be difficult to diagnose accurately and manage. This may happen if the occlusal vertical dimension is excessive, meaning that the denture bearing area is perpetually overloaded. Leaving one or both dentures out can help to confirm the diagnosis. This type of pain can also present if there is an allergy or an intolerance to materials in the denture base. If this is suspected, it will be important to send the patient for patch testing for sensitivity to denture-base materials.

• *Immediate intolerance* – It is always a concern when the patient is unable to retain a prosthesis in the mouth for any time at all. Occasionally this may be because of acute trauma from the prostheses, making fully seating them painful. However, it is often the case that patients are reluctant to insert their prostheses – and begin to reject them before they are even fully inserted into the mouth. This rejection may also be accompanied with a gag reflex, which is discussed further below. There are often psychosocial problems that will complicate the acceptance of a removable prosthesis and it is important that the patient feels comfortable enough to highlight any concerns. You must also be sensitive to the fact that some patients may have experienced traumatic events in the past that have manifested as oral intolerances. Be prepared on some occasions to refer patients, via their general practitioner, for counselling.

• *Received multiple consecutive sets* – Patients that present with a bag full of previous dentures should be assessed very carefully. The previously failed prostheses are usually a warning sign that risk factors have been missed – it is also often the case that patient expectations have been mismanaged. In this case, just assess the set of dentures that the patient prefers or wears most frequently.

• *Lack of recent prosthetic experience* – Patients presenting without any dentures, or who have not been wearing any recently, must be informed that the acclimatisation process will necessarily be longer. It also makes prescribing the tooth positions and the vertical dimension more challenging.

• *History of non-perseverance* – If patients are unable or unwilling to persevere in order to overcome minor problems with their prostheses, then it is likely that the prognosis will be significantly affected.

• *Poor neuromuscular control or dexterity* – If the patient has suffered a stroke, or has been diagnosed with Parkinson's disease or other neuromuscular disorders, then the prognosis will be significantly affected.

Clinical factors

The following clinical factors can significantly compromise the outcome of denture provision:

- Restricted intraoral access
- Dry mouth
- Widespread or significant ulceration (especially if the patient is taking nicorandil)
- A gag reflex when the DBA is palpated
- Obvious hyperactivity of the tongue or lateral tongue spread
- Superficial mental nerves causing pain on palpation
- Significant tori that will impede extension or full seating of a prosthesis
- A large discrepancy between the current intercuspal position and the retruded arc of closure
- Problems or difficulties with the patient's ability to sit upright in a dental chair

Ridge anatomy

It is generally accepted that an atrophic ridge means that the prognosis will be affected, especially on the lower arch. In these cases, more attention needs to be paid to accurate extensions, functional border moulding and tooth position. However, it is often assumed that high and rounded ridges means a high chance of 'success' – but be careful – patients with ridges of this type often present with pain on the crest of the ridge. Ridges should also be inspected for the height of the muscle attachments – are they near the crest of the ridge (which means you need to be very careful to accommodate them in function) or are they low or absent? Also look for significant ridge undercuts, which may mean that you need to consider a specific path of insertion, or even pre-prosthetic surgery.

Technical factors

Poor communication with the laboratory means that technical aspects may be suboptimal. Make it clear on your communications to the laboratory why you are making the prostheses and ask the technician to contact you if they encounter any problems or suboptimal clinical work.

Ultimately, success is compromised by poor communication between operator, patient and technician – be honest about your likelihood of success and document the discussions carefully in the patient notes.

8 Accessibility and operator position

Figure 8.1 Accessibility and operator position

Upper arch

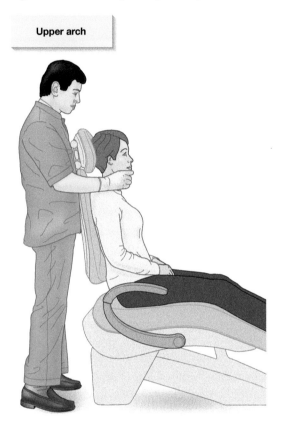

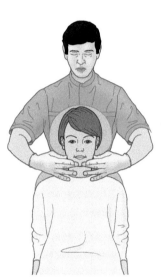

- Straight back behind the patient
- Allows stability of posture
- Allows support for the patient's head
- Allows control of the mandible and peri-oral area
- Allows correct manipulation and seating of the trays

Tray handles

- Control
- Orientation
- Allow material to fully engage relevant holes and grooves

Lower arch

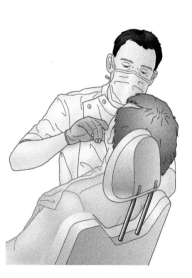

- Sitting or standing in front of the patient
- Straight back
- Allows correct manipulation and seating of the trays
- Allows optimal field of direct vision
- Improves inter-arch visibility, especially posteriorly

Removable Prosthodontics at a Glance, First Edition. James Field and Claire Storey. © 2020 James Field and Claire Storey. Published 2020 by John Wiley & Sons Ltd.
Companion Website: www.wiley.com/go/field/removable

Successful clinical stages during prosthetic treatment are not just dependent on your technical ability. The previous chapter talked about how limited intraoral access, or the inability of the patient to sit in your dental chair, are risk factors for failure. However, it is equally as important to consider your *posture* and *operating position*.

Posture and operating position

It is easy to forget your posture when you are concentrating on a clinical stage. Some types of saddle seat, or wearing loupes, can help to reinforce a good posture – however, with the exception of tooth preparations, we would recommend carrying out each prosthodontic clinic stage in a standing position.

Maintaining a dynamic position around the patient means that you are less likely to strain your neck or back, and more likely to move into an appropriate position. This will ensure that your back and neck will remain healthy, and your operative dental career will be more sustainable! Aside from your own health, it is also more comfortable for patients to have impressions taken when they are sitting upright rather than in the supine position.

Move yourself, and the patient

A dynamic operating position means that you are able to move yourself around the patient, but that you are also moving the patient into an appropriate position. Typically as dentists we are good at neither, often staying around the 12 o'clock operator position. It is very important to make sure that you are comfortable first, before considering how you can then move the patient to optimise your field of view or operative control. This may mean moving the patient up or down in the chair, reclining the patient or simply turning their head to either side. Ensure that wherever possible you maintain a straight back, straight neck and direct vision of the operative area.

Upper arches

Typically we would recommend operating from behind the patient when working on impressions for the upper arch (Figure 8.1). You should stand with the top of the patient's head at the level of your non-dominant elbow. Do not stand immediately behind the patient – instead, imagine that you are holding the patient's head like a rugby ball, or that you are getting them into a 'head lock' – so slightly to the side. When your hands meet in front of the patient's mouth, your hands should be lower than your elbows. Imagine water running down your arms, and off your little fingertips – the 'first position' in ballet. This position serves a multitude of functions:
• Ensures that you are able to stand with a straight back
• Ensures stability of posture so that you can manipulate the patient confidently and securely
• Allows you to support the patient's head with your non-dominant arm
• Gives you control of the mandibular lower border, should you need to encourage the patient into a particular position
• Gives you control of the perioral area (which is especially useful if the patient has a habit of raising their hands to reach for their mouth)

• Allows you to palpate and inspect the full upper denture-bearing area
• Facilitates the correct manipulation and seating of trays because of a greater range of wrist movements (trying to fully seat an upper tray, posterior aspect first, from in front of the patient is incredibly difficult)

Lower arches

In most cases we would recommend making impressions of the lower arch from in front of the patient, with the patient sitting upright (Figure 8.2). Most dental chairs become narrower halfway down, and this is a good place to position yourself. Ensure you have a straight back, rather than allowing yourself to bend over forwards. One of the aspects of lower special trays that is most poorly extended and adapted is the labial extension. This is often because operators are sitting behind the patient when assessing this area, which results in inappropriate manipulation of the lower lip. Once again, your arms should not be raised – instead, they should adopt a similar position to that described for an upper arch position. Dental chairs tend to need to be lowered considerably to achieve this position. However, it is also useful for the following reasons:
• Facilitates the correct manipulation and seating of trays because of a greater range of wrist movements
• Field of view is not blocked by the facial anatomy, which causes operators behind the patient to lean forwards
• Encourages a straight back
• Improves interarch visibility for assessing occlusal relationships, facial aesthetics and speech

Control of the prostheses and trays

It is very important that you take control of inserting and removing impression trays, and the patient's prostheses. When *you* insert and remove prostheses, you are able to look closely at the way in which the extensions and fitting surface engage with the tissues, and check paths of insertion. You are also able to apply appropriate pressure to certain areas in order to check stability or painful trigger points. If the *patient* continually removes and inserts their prostheses, then they often take the opportunity to displace them in fairly imaginative ways – and it is these parafunctional habits that you will spend much of your time counselling them against. Further, in relation to impressions – never leave an impression in the patient's mouth without being in full control. This means not letting go and performing another task – and handles are critically important in ensuring control, tray orientation and efficient and effective removal.

Other considerations

Restricted access might mean that you need to use a syringe to deliver material onto the denture-bearing anatomy and then insert the tray as the carrier. When rotating trays into the mouth, it is useful to ask the patient to 'half close' – and applying Vaseline to the corners of the mouth can avoid trauma to friable tissues.

9 Pre-prosthetic treatment

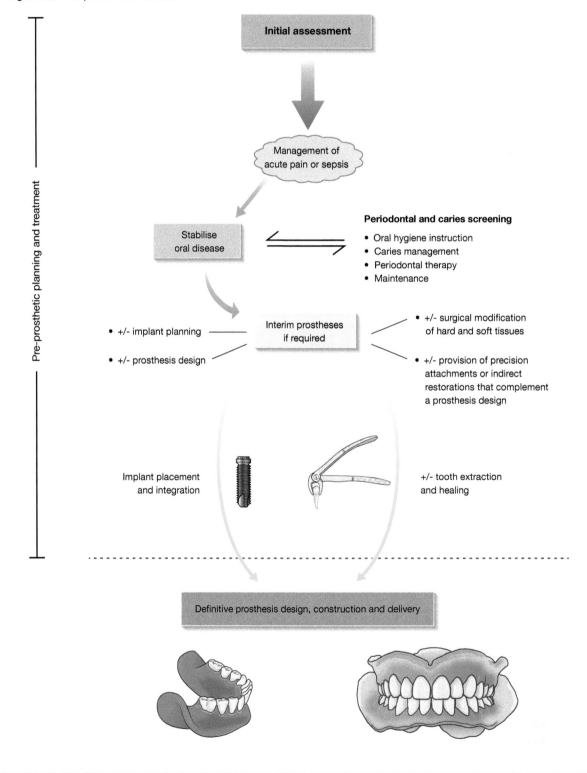

Figure 9.1 Pre-prosthetic treatment

Pre-prosthetic planning and treatment

Initial assessment

Management of acute pain or sepsis

Stabilise oral disease

Periodontal and caries screening
• Oral hygiene instruction
• Caries management
• Periodontal therapy
• Maintenance

• +/- implant planning
• +/- prosthesis design

Interim prostheses if required

• +/- surgical modification of hard and soft tissues

• +/- provision of precision attachments or indirect restorations that complement a prosthesis design

Implant placement and integration

+/- tooth extraction and healing

Definitive prosthesis design, construction and delivery

Removable Prosthodontics at a Glance, First Edition. James Field and Claire Storey. © 2020 James Field and Claire Storey. Published 2020 by John Wiley & Sons Ltd.
Companion Website: www.wiley.com/go/field/removable

When embarking upon the provision of removable prostheses, it is important to assess the patient's oral environment comprehensively. Achieving a stable foundation is the bedrock upon which successful rehabilitation will be built. Castles cannot be built on sand. *Pre-prosthetic treatment* involves the care that is delivered *prior* to the planning and delivery of prostheses (Figure 9.1). This may involve:
• Management of acute pain/sepsis
• Stabilisation of any active oral disease including periodontal disease, caries, soft tissue conditions and neoplasia
• Surgical modification of hard and soft tissues to facilitate retention and/or stability of the prosthesis

Extraoral assessment

A careful extraoral assessment can reveal the following features, which may impact on how and when you provide prosthetic rehabilitation:
• Facial asymmetries
• Skeletal class
• Restrictions or trismus
• Hypertrophy of muscles of mastication
• Degree of mobility and dexterity

Edentulous patients

Where the fully edentulous patient is concerned, the condition of the soft tissues should be assessed and the architecture of the bony hard and overlying soft tissues noted. This was discussed in Chapter 4 – however, it is important to note that significant undercuts, tori, or fibrous tissue may benefit from pre-prosthetic surgery. It may also be the case that muscle attachments may need repositioning, vestibules surgically deepened, sharp ridges smoothed, keratinised tissues augmented and previous surgical sites debulked. The latter are often carried out in conjunction with oral surgeons – and any pre-prosthetic surgery will need to be consented and planned appropriately, with a suitable period of healing prior to provision of the definitive prosthesis. Consideration should be given for how the patient will manage in the interim, either without a prosthesis in place, or by making modifications to existing ones.

Partially dentate patients

Where the partially dentate patient is concerned, additional observations must be made around the condition of the remaining dentition including:
• Active dental disease (plaque control, caries and periodontal health)
• Type of occlusion including any evidence of bruxism or parafunction
• Limitations caused by drifted, overerupted and tilted teeth
• Endodontic status of teeth
• Status of any existing direct or indirect restorations

Periodontal disease and caries

Where teeth have been lost because of periodontal disease, a thorough assessment of periodontal health including a basic periodontal examination (BPE) should be carried out. When a code 3 or 4 presents, a personalised prevention programme should be instigated and suitably demonstrated by the clinician. If a code 4 persists (pocketing above 5.5 mm after plaque control has been optimised and superficial inflammation resolved), then full mouth 6-point pocket charting should be completed. For persistent deep and bleeding pockets, a course of non-surgical management should be undertaken, supported by regular full mouth disclosed plaque and bleeding scores. Subgingival instrumentation should utilise local anaesthesia to comfortably treat deeper and inflamed periodontal pockets, or where tooth sensitivity causes patient distress. Ultrasonic debridement is recommended for this as an effective and efficient method, whilst preventing excessive cementum removal. The 6-point pocket charting should be reassessed 2–3 months following treatment. Generally, periodontal health may be assumed when bleeding is at fewer than 10% of sites and pocket probing depths are no greater than 4 mm, with no bleeding at the 4 mm deep sites.

During periodontal stabilisation treatment, the patient may need to have teeth extracted that are deemed of hopeless prognosis, especially if they present as lone standing and grade III mobile, have bone loss progressing towards the tooth apex (or a true perio-endo lesion), or have been unresponsive to periodontal treatment. During this stabilisation phase a temporary acrylic denture may need to be provided to restore aesthetics and masticatory function, and to reduce occlusal trauma on remaining tooth units. The prosthesis is likely to be entirely mucosa borne, and so care should be taken with the design to ensure that trauma at the gingival margins because of denture displacement is avoided. The contact points between the saddles and abutment teeth should be cleansable, and the patient should be counselled with respect to plaque control on the denture and on the abutment teeth. Even a well-polished acrylic denture acts as a bacterial reservoir and it is for this reason that in short span rehabilitations, resin-bonded bridgework should be considered as an alternative in order to minimise plaque retention; this clearly depends on the quality of the abutment teeth.

Appropriate prevention with diet counselling, hygiene and fluoride therapy should be instigated where the caries risk is raised. Where conservation work is required, this can also allow for construction of restorations which aid the support and retention of the final removable partial denture. Restorations (both direct and indirect) can be fabricated with rest seats, guide planes, adequate bulbosities and precision elements to aid the success of the denture. Accurate primary impressions and mounted study models are essential planning aids for the prosthetic rehabilitation. Aesthetics can also be assessed and addressed at this stage, considering modifications such as composite augmentation to correct tooth dimensions and paths of insertion for minimising dead spaces.

Implants

Implants may well form part of definitive pre-prosthodontic treatment. Restoratively driven assessment, case selection and planning are essential in order to maximise success. Following the stabilisation of existing oral disease, an optimised prosthesis should be constructed in order to assess aesthetic and functional acceptability and define the ideal prosthetic envelope. This can help to plan the implant positions and trajectories. The restoration of two mandibular parasymphyseal implants with overdenture abutments is discussed in Chapter 41.

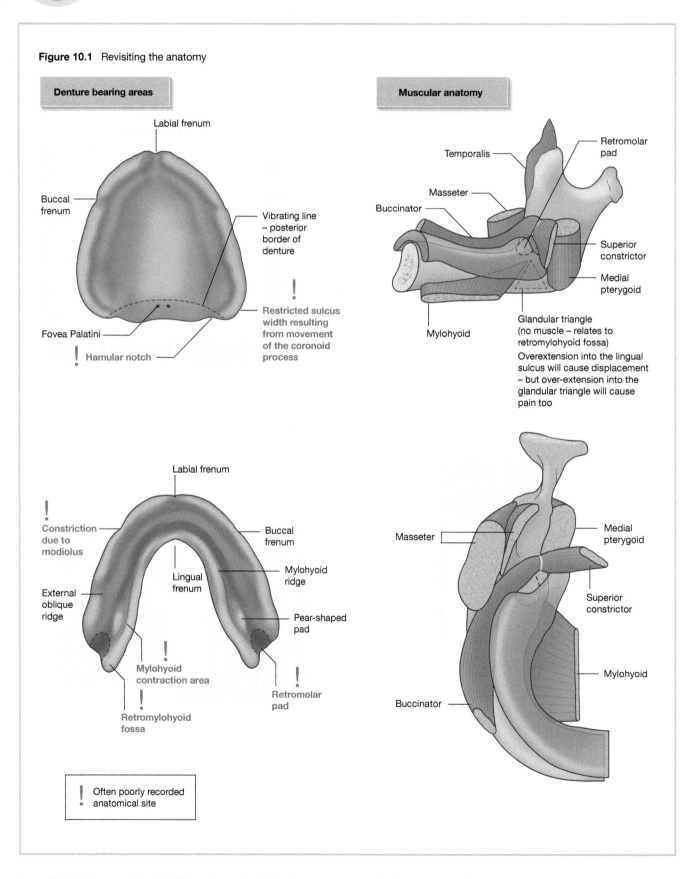

10 # Revisiting the anatomy

Figure 10.1 Revisiting the anatomy

Denture bearing areas

Labial frenum

Buccal frenum

Vibrating line – posterior border of denture

! Restricted sulcus width resulting from movement of the coronoid process

Fovea Palatini

! Hamular notch

Muscular anatomy

Temporalis

Retromolar pad

Masseter

Buccinator

Superior constrictor

Medial pterygoid

Mylohyoid

Glandular triangle (no muscle – relates to retromylohyoid fossa)
Overextension into the lingual sulcus will cause displacement – but over-extension into the glandular triangle will cause pain too

Labial frenum

! Constriction due to modiolus

Buccal frenum

Lingual frenum

Mylohyoid ridge

External oblique ridge

Pear-shaped pad

! Mylohyoid contraction area

! Retromolar pad

! Retromylohyoid fossa

Masseter

Medial pterygoid

Superior constrictor

Mylohyoid

Buccinator

! Often poorly recorded
■ anatomical site

Removable Prosthodontics at a Glance, First Edition. James Field and Claire Storey. © 2020 James Field and Claire Storey. Published 2020 by John Wiley & Sons Ltd.
Companion Website: www.wiley.com/go/field/removable

t is very easy to forget the denture-bearing anatomy. In the end, we tend to focus only on the ridge form, noting whether it is rounded, or flat and atrophic. Perhaps attention may also be paid to whether there are any fibrous (or flabby) aspects of the ridge (Chapter 17).

In actual fact, there is a need to recall the full denture-bearing and limiting anatomy – not least so the current status quo can be accurately assessed – but clearly a working knowledge of the anatomy is important for obtaining accurate functional impressions. For this reason it is also important to be aware of muscle movements which allow the limiting anatomy to be accurately recorded – and these will be discussed further, below (Figure 10.1).

Upper arch

The upper arch is probably the simplest in terms of identifiable anatomic structures – and yet many dentures that are constructed fail to respect much of the anatomy. Whilst most of us will correctly identify frenal attachments, it is important to consider whether these have a relatively high or a low attachment to the edentulous ridge. This will indicate how carefully you will need to adjust the special trays, and how significantly the finished denture base will deviate from the general sulcal depth in that area. Overextension around frenal attachments is still, however, very common.

The fovea palatini sit, most frequently, around 3–4 mm posterior to the vibrating line (the junction between the hard and soft palate). It is important to identify this junction, because this marks the optimal posterior border of the upper denture. We will discuss later the technical importance of the vibrating line and how it aids in developing a border seal.

Two pieces of anatomy that are very frequently neglected are:
1 The restrictions created by the coronoid process when mandibular excursions occur. Try placing your index finger in your upper buccal sulcus and extend it along to the second molar. Try moving your jaw left and right! It is necessary to *encourage lateral mandibular movements* during the working impression in order to accurately record these restrictions, otherwise the patient will experience pain, or dislodgement of the denture.
2 The hamular notches, which represent the posterior border of the tuberosity joining the medial and lateral plates of the pterygoid process. This is primarily because of the fact that materials chosen for working impressions are not supported sufficiently by a well-extended tray. It is also necessary to *encourage and manipulate impression materials* around *the tuberosities and the hamular notches* in order to develop a strong border seal. This will be covered later in Chapter 15.

Lower arch

The lower arch is often complicated by several factors:
• The tongue and its lateral spread and possible hyperactivity
• The challenge of defining the limited anatomy on an atrophic ridge

• Potential lingual undercuts or mandibular tori
• The action of several relatively deep and complex muscles, which cannot be activated independently

It is very important *before* you pick up a stock tray, or indeed a special tray, to remind yourself of the obvious limiting anatomy of the lower arch. Asking the patient to *lift their tongue*, gives an immediate idea of tongue spread, frenal attachments and lingual sulcal depth. Asking the patient to *relax the lower lip as you gently lift it upward* to reveal the true functional sulcus depth is also a very useful exercise. Often on atrophic ridges, virtually no functional sulcus remains. You should be mindful of this, when adjusting the special trays and taking the working impression. Gently *reflecting the buccal mucosa* around the entire arch can give you a good visual representation of the ridge anatomy and help to identify the external oblique ridge, which represents the main bearing area of the lower denture. Palpating this area can help too. Other limiting anatomy that is commonly unaccounted for is discussed below.

Anterior limiting anatomy

Aside from the labial sulcus discussed above, *Modiolus* is a complex confluence of perioral muscles (buccinator, orbicularis oris, levator and depressor muscles, risorius, platysma and zygomaticus major) that meet slightly lateral to the corner of the mouth. If activation of these muscles is not accounted for, then the lower denture base can become perpetually antero-posteriorly and superficially displaced during speech, mastication and facial expression. It is an extremely variable piece of anatomy and so asking patients to employ certain movements is the best way to record this limiting anatomy. This will be discussed further in Chapter 16.

Posterior limiting anatomy

In order for a border seal to be established on the lower arch, it is necessary to account for the insertions of buccinators distally. Stock trays can indiscriminately overextend the special tray buccally and so careful tray adjustment is advised. The lower denture should sit over the keratinised pear-shaped pad (representing the scar tissue from the last standing molar) and up onto the retromolar pad. Full coverage of the retromolar pad is not advised – primarily, because this tissue is only para-keratinised and glandular (and so it does not contribute significantly to denture stability) – but also because extension in this area can complicate later stages with heel clash of the denture bases.

Medial limiting anatomy

The lingual sulcus is notoriously difficult to respect – and extreme tongue movements can help to activate this anatomy. In particular, palatoglossus is the only muscle that will elevate the posterior tongue *and* maintain the palatoglossal arch (which retains saliva in the mouth) – this, and mylohyoid (which defines and reinforces the floor of the mouth), can only be activated by swallowing and speaking. Tongue movements that record the full limiting anatomy will be discussed in Chapter 16.

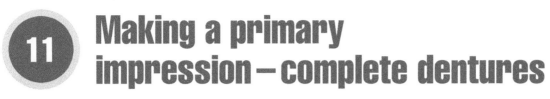

11 Making a primary impression – complete dentures

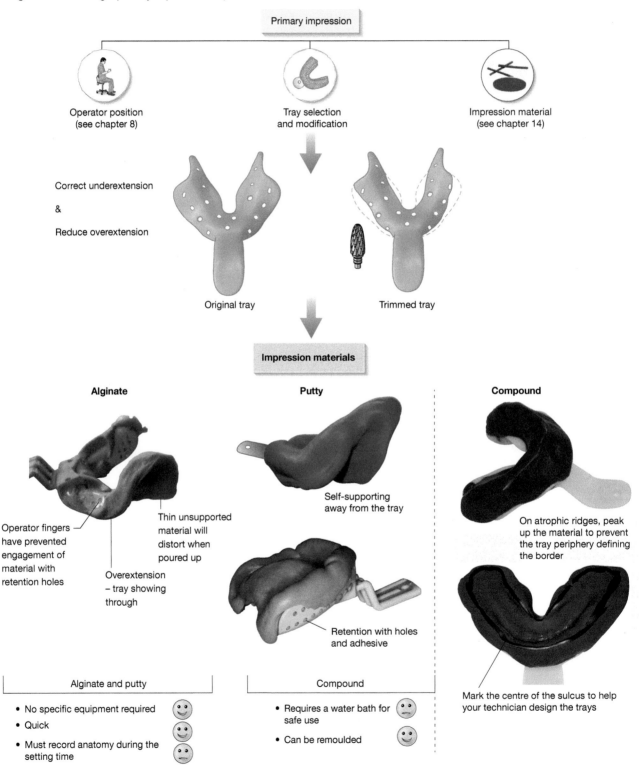

Figure 11.1 Making a primary impression for partial dentures

Primary impression

Operator position
(see chapter 8)

Tray selection
and modification

Impression material
(see chapter 14)

Correct underextension

&

Reduce overextension

Original tray

Trimmed tray

Impression materials

Alginate

Operator fingers
have prevented
engagement of
material with
retention holes

Thin unsupported
material will
distort when
poured up

Overextension
– tray showing
through

Putty

Self-supporting
away from the tray

Retention with holes
and adhesive

Compound

On atrophic ridges, peak
up the material to prevent
the tray periphery defining
the border

Mark the centre of the sulcus to help
your technician design the trays

Alginate and putty

- No specific equipment required
- Quick
- Must record anatomy during the setting time

Compound

- Requires a water bath for safe use
- Can be remoulded

Removable Prosthodontics at a Glance, First Edition. James Field and Claire Storey. © 2020 James Field and Claire Storey. Published 2020 by John Wiley & Sons Ltd.
Companion Website: www.wiley.com/go/field/removable

The assumption is often made that primary impressions for complete dentures do not really need to 'do that much'. I often hear people saying, 'I'll get a proper impression once my special tray comes back'. In fact, the primary impressions are one of the most critical stages of complete denture construction and underpin the remainder of the clinical and technical stages.

Primary impressions for complete dentures should:

- Record the full denture-bearing area
- Capture the *functional* sulcus depth
- Ideally account for any limiting anatomy
- Show no voids, drags or air blows
- Show no tears or detachment from the tray
- Be central in the tray with an even thickness of material

This will allow an accurate special tray to be made that requires minimal adjustment and will record the anatomy in function. Making the effort at this stage pays dividends later both in terms of accuracy and time. A good primary impression is influenced by (i) operator position (already discussed in Chapter 8), (ii) the tray and (iii) the impression material

Choice of tray

Most edentulous stock trays on the upper arch are a reasonable starting point for primary impressions. Use the patient's existing dentures as a guide in order to help select the correct size of tray. The lower arch tends to be more problematic and using the existing denture as a guide (especially if they are underextended distally) will lead to inaccuracies. Atrophic ridges can further complicate using a lower stock tray – so do not be afraid to trim the trays before you begin (see Figure 11.1). Otherwise, the special trays will often come back very overextended in the labial and lingual sulcus and require significant adjustment.

Material

There is a lot of debate about which material provides the best outcomes for primary impressions. If you are confident about handling the material, and you have reasonably adapted trays, then it probably makes little difference – however, it is important to understand the limitations of the different available materials and to choose one that works best in your hands. The three main choices of material are discussed below.

1 *Alginate* is a cheap and quick material to use. However, it is unable to support itself in thin section and is therefore poor at recording anatomy that is more than a few millimetres from the tray periphery. Typically, this means that distal aspects on the upper, and disto-lingual aspects on the lower, are poorly recorded. Alginate is also easily displaced from the tray border, meaning that the material is more likely to begin to lift or peel away from the tray. Finally, alginate is not stiff and is unable to resist distortion when it is poured with plaster (which is heavy). Alginate that is not supported by a tray will distort, and you will be none the wiser. If you have ever had a special tray that seems to adapt to the ridge anteriorly, but has a larger discrepancy posteriorly, then that is most probably why. Some clinicians advocate a two-stage alginate primary impression in order to overcome some of these apparent problems. An initial impression is taken, which is then cut back at the periphery. A final wash impression is then taken, which allows the alginate to more reliably record distant anatomy. Whilst this is often true, there still tends to be a poor record of the full aspects of the tuberosities and the hamular notches.

2 *Impression compound* has been considered the gold standard within teaching hospitals for many years, because it is thought to give the most predictable and stable impression and can be reliably disinfected. This material must be heated to 56 °C in order for it to reach its glass transition temperature. At this point it is mouldable, but importantly it will also support itself independently from the tray. It is possible to rewarm and remould compound several times and so this can be an excellent material of choice for difficult cases. The drawback is that ideally a water-bath should be used in order to temper the material to the correct temperature and to prevent it cooling down. Once a relatively thick amount of compound has cooled, it takes a disproportionately long time to warm it up again. The viscosity of compound (in contrast to alginate) also means that it is common to over-record relatively shallow sulci, such as the lower labial segment. In this case, it is possible, after disinfection, to demarcate the sulcal anatomy so that the technician knows where to extend the special trays (see Figure 11.1).

3 *Silicone putty* provides a happy medium, in my opinion (not laboratory putty, which is not licensed for intraoral use). Quick and easy to manipulate, clinical putty offers benefits common to both compound and alginate. However, there is a defined working time, and once the material has set, it cannot easily be modified. It does, however, provide a resilient and robust primary impression, which can be poured-up with accuracy. Putty has a tendency to drag, and so it is important to encourage the putty back up against the tray in areas where this is likely to happen, such as around the tuberosities or the distal extensions of the lower arch.

Lower arches

Both compound and silicone putty allow the material to be 'built-up' in the tray prior to taking the impression (see Figure 11.1) which can help to record the ridge and sulcal anatomy without having to fully seat the tray. This means that the tray extensions are less likely to over-record the limiting anatomy. It is also tempting to 'pinch' the lower tray against the lower border of the mandible, between thumb and forefinger. However, you *should* just use the tray handle to hold the tray in place, otherwise the material fails to engage the retentive slots or holes (see Figure 11.1); this approach also prevents the trays from digging into the lateral aspects of the ridges.

If the arch is not central in the tray, or the ridges are too close to the tray edges, then you will feel resistance and assume that the tray is fully seated, when it is not.

Finally, once the impression has been checked and disinfected, you must inform the technician of your choice of wash material so that the correct thickness of spacer is employed. This is discussed further in Chapter 13.

Making a primary impression – partial dentures

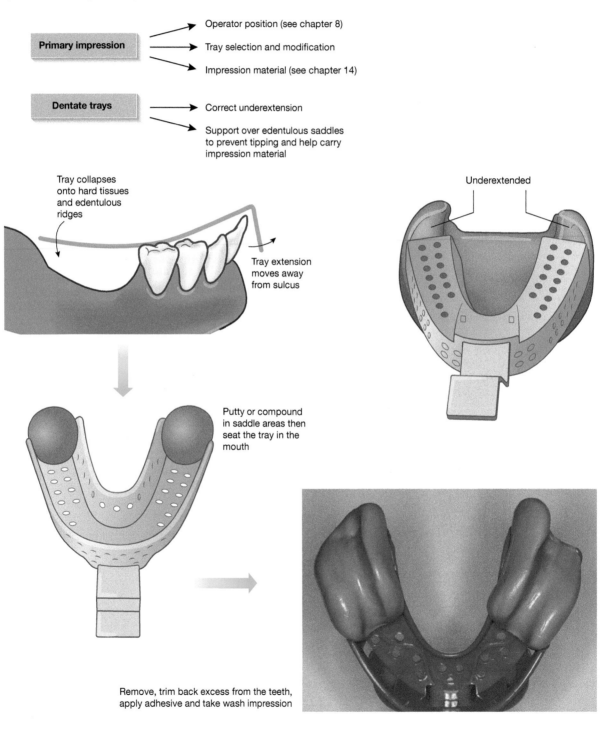

Figure 12.1 Making a primary impression for partial prostheses

Primary impression
→ Operator position (see chapter 8)
→ Tray selection and modification
→ Impression material (see chapter 14)

Dentate trays
→ Correct underextension
→ Support over edentulous saddles to prevent tipping and help carry impression material

Tray collapses onto hard tissues and edentulous ridges

Tray extension moves away from sulcus

Underextended

Putty or compound in saddle areas then seat the tray in the mouth

Remove, trim back excess from the teeth, apply adhesive and take wash impression

Removable Prosthodontics at a Glance, First Edition. James Field and Claire Storey. © 2020 James Field and Claire Storey. Published 2020 by John Wiley & Sons Ltd.
Companion Website: www.wiley.com/go/field/removable

As described in Chapter 13, primary impressions underpin the remainder of the clinical and technical stages. A well-made primary impression will ensure that the special tray is well extended and that the prosthesis covers the full denture-bearing area (DBA). This concept is often overlooked when taking impressions of partially dentate arches. This is especially the case when elements of direct retention are also employed, such as denture clasps, implants and extracoronal attachments. In reality, utilising the full DBA is equally as important in order to ensure that support is truly mucosa- and toothborne – and to avoid relying too heavily on mechanical elements, which will otherwise undoubtedly perish sooner.

Primary impressions for partially dentate arches should:

- Record the full remaining dentition and DBA
- Capture the functional sulcus depth
- Ideally account for any limiting anatomy
- Show no voids, drags or air blows
- Show no tears or detachment from the tray
- Be central in the tray with an even thickness of material

Choice of tray

The recording of edentulous ridges in partially dentate patients is complicated by the fact that we are forced to use dentate trays. There is significant potential with free-end saddles for trays to tip onto the edentulous ridges if they are not supported – as the tray rotates it complicates accurate recording of the lingual or labial sulcus. Further, dentate trays do not often reach the full DBA (see Figure 12.1).

Conversely, dentate trays may occasionally need significant adjustment in order to account for displaced teeth, or particularly shallow sulci. Take the time to ensure that the tray fits the arch form.

Sometimes a smaller tray is an adequate length, but just needs to be slightly wider. A larger tray is either difficult to insert or extends too far posteriorly. In this case, it is possible to modify most commercial plastic/acrylic trays by heating in the midline with a flame or hot air burner. Once warmed, the tray can be expanded before being cooled and retried in the mouth. Some commercial primary trays are designed to be heated and modified, although this feature often attracts a premium price.

Finally, inserting a loaded dentate tray into the mouth can be particularly challenging. They are inevitably deeper than the equivalent edentulous trays, and it is important to check that you are in a suitable operator position. The patient should be relaxed and 'half-close' whilst you rotate the impression tray into the mouth. One hand should retract the soft tissue of the cheek whilst the other hand rotates the tray into the mouth on the opposite side. Do not begin to seat the tray until you are sure that the antero-posterior position is correct. Seat the heels first, to ensure that excess material is displaced anteriorly along the sulcus, and keep the lip retracted until the tray is fully seated.

Material

The presence of teeth, and associated undercuts, limits the choice of impression materials available for partial impressions.

Whichever material is used to record the teeth, it is almost always the case, especially with free-end saddles, or saddles greater than about 2 cm, that a supportive material is required to effectively stabilise the tray and carry wash material to the distant anatomy. The main choices of supportive and impression material are discussed below.

Supportive materials

Both impression compound and clinical putty provide excellent support over edentulous saddles in partially dentate arches. They also act effectively to extend the tray in free-end saddles or around maxillary tuberosities, ensuring that the impression material is not unsupported. The merits and drawbacks of each material are described in Chapter 14. Given that these materials act only to support a less viscous material, clinical putty tends to be the most practical solution. A small amount of putty is mixed and placed into the dentate tray over the edentulous areas (Figure 12.1). The tray is seated for a moment whilst the putty firms, taking care not to allow the tray bottom to touch the occlusal or incisal surfaces. The tray is removed and putty that has been in contact with the hard tissues is removed with a wax knife or a scalpel. Once set, this can be retried in the mouth in order to practise fully seating the tray. The actual impression can then be taken over the top in order to record the dentate areas accurately.

Impression materials

A number of materials can be used to take the definitive impression. These are outlined below. Regardless, a suitable adhesive should be used to ensure that the impression material binds to the supportive material and the exposed tray. At this point, it is vital to ensure that the impression material is not overloaded onto the tray. It is common for this to happen, but it means that you will often fail to fully seat the tray – and in this circumstance you are essentially using an unmodified stock tray once again. Remember that the impression material should be elastic, otherwise you will be unable to remove the impression from the undercuts around the teeth. Zinc oxide eugenol is therefore contraindicated in this situation.

Alginate is a cheap, quick and effective material to use for this purpose. If you notice large undercuts or multiple embrasure spaces, then alginate will tend to tear. In these circumstances it is worth considering a more resilient material like silicone.

Silicones (light- or medium-bodied) are more expensive but are more accurately applied to the impression tray. The working time is slightly longer, allowing you to ensure that the tray is fully seated, and that you have time to carry out some basic functional border moulding.

As always, once the impression has been checked and disinfected, you must prescribe your intended wash material for the working impression to the technician. This way, they can employ the correct thickness of spacer when constructing the special tray. This is discussed further in Chapter 13.

13 Special trays

Figure 13.1 Special trays

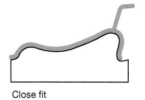

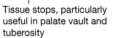
Special trays

• Should have the amount of spacer prescribed, with or without tissue stops

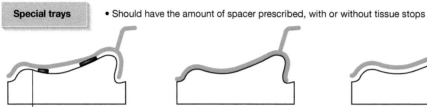

Tissue stops, particularly useful in palate vault and tuberosity

Close fit

Classic spaced

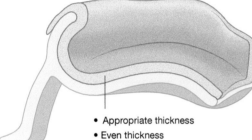

• Appropriate thickness
• Even thickness
• Supported by the tray

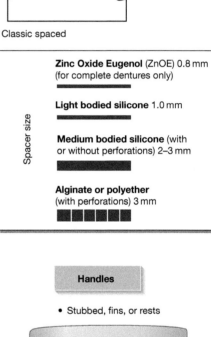

Spacer size

Zinc Oxide Eugenol (ZnOE) 0.8 mm (for complete dentures only)

Light bodied silicone 1.0 mm

Medium bodied silicone (with or without perforations) 2–3 mm

Alginate or polyether (with perforations) 3 mm

Extensions

• Accuracy depends on the primary impressions
• May require trimming
• Check in the mouth not on the casts

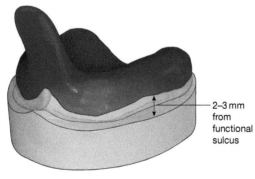

2–3 mm from functional sulcus

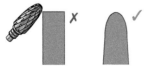

✗   ✓

Handles

• Stubbed, fins, or rests

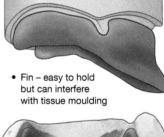

• Fin – easy to hold but can interfere with tissue moulding

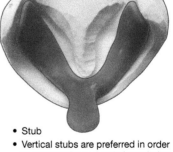

• Stub
• Vertical stubs are preferred in order to prevent tissue restrictions during border moulding

onstruction of a special (or custom) tray is often a crucial stage of the denture-making process. The special tray should allow relatively close adaptation to the full denture-bearing area, so that an accurate and functional impression can be obtained. Of course, the extensions of the special tray are dependent on the anatomy picked up in the primary impression; there is little point asking for a special tray to be made if it will require significant modification at the chairside. The less accurate the primary impression, the less 'special or custom' the subsequent tray can be.

Ideally the special tray will allow an impression to be made which is sympathetic to the impression material, allowing a suitable and uniform thickness of material between the tray and the denture-bearing anatomy. Tray extensions should sit 2–3 mm from the base of the functional sulcus – the methods to determine this will be discussed in Chapters 15 and 16. However, tray extensions should *not* be assessed by sitting the tray on the primary cast. Regardless of how the tray is constructed or adjusted, it should have smooth and rounded peripheries. A carbide acrylic bur (shaped like a gherkin) should be used to adjust the periphery of trays (Figure 13.1).

Materials

Most special trays are constructed with sheets of light-cured resin or shellac, a thermoplastic material. Light-cured resin trays often present with an uncured surface layer (the oxygen-inhibited layer), which should be removed by the laboratory prior to tray use. This uncured layer should not come into contact with soft tissues. For this reason, it is also very important to wear gloves when handling light-cured acrylic trays. When adjusting the trays at the chairside, it is important to remember that acrylic dust should be suctioned away immediately with a high-volume aspirator to ensure that it is not inhaled by those nearby – this is to avoid the risk of silicosis. Trimmed trays should also be rinsed in order to avoid the transfer of resin dust or unpolymerised resin to the soft tissues. Whilst shellac does not create dust particulate, it often melts with the heat of the straight hand piece bur, which can be uncomfortable if it comes into near contact with skin.

Tray spacers and tissue stops

Depending on your choice of impression material, the laboratory may introduce a tray spacer between the cast and your special tray. This is routinely prescribed for relatively viscous materials, and it ensures that hydrostatic pressure is minimised, whilst allowing the material to flow across the full anatomical area. The following spacers are often prescribed:

- Zinc oxide eugenol (ZnOE) – 0.8 mm
- Alginate – 3 mm
- Light-bodied silicone – 1 mm
- Medium-bodied silicone – 2–3 mm

Some laboratories leave no spacer at all for ZnOE. In this case, it can be very useful to employ tissue stops. Tissue stops help to ensure an even thickness of impression material, by preventing over-seating of the tray in any particular area (Figure 13.1). Tissue stops can be fabricated by the laboratory, or at the chairside. It is easiest to ask the laboratory to create these for you, but if you

are fabricating them at the chairside, I would recommend a relatively rigid material such as greenstick, impression compound or clinical putty. These should be fashioned by gently seating the tray in the mouth to the intended depth and then trimming back any excess material from the stops. Aim to place them in supportive areas, such as over ridges and in the palate.

Handles

Tray handles should be designed and positioned so that you can adequately control the tray, whilst at the same time allowing free movement of the local soft tissues. A small, vertical handle, sitting over the crest of the edentulous ridge, is often the best type. Larger, broader handles can interfere with border moulding.

Sometimes auxiliary handles or handles in alternative positions are added – this might be to allow pick-up impressions for implants, to allow windowing of a tray, or simply to provide more even load distribution over the entire ridge. It is a good idea to inform the laboratory where you would like the handles to be placed – especially if it deviates from your normal requirements.

Material retention and support

As mentioned previously, it is incredibly important that primary *and* working impressions are fully supported by the tray, otherwise the impression is likely to distort when poured with gypsum products, which are heavy. It is very difficult to determine whether this has happened or not. That said, it is equally as important to ensure that impression materials do no peel away or detach from the impression tray – otherwise pouring the models will also create an invisible distortion. There are two main methods to ensure that this detachment is minimised – (i) the use of adhesives, and (ii) mechanical tray features (such as perforation holes, slots or rim locks).

- *Adhesives* – Often tray adhesives contain hazardous chemicals such as xylenes, siloxanes and benzene – accordingly, trays should be tried in the mouth, and adjusted, *prior* to adhesives being applied. A thin and uniform coat should be applied, which is then air-dried prior to application of the impression material. It is important to ensure that the adhesive reaches the full periphery of the tray, including sulcal extensions. A paper sheet underneath the tray can help to contain stray aerosol or drips from brush-based products. Cross-infection control is paramount. For brush-based products, these should be first dispensed into a Dappen dish prior to application onto the tray.
- *Perforations* – Perforations are often used for less close-fitting trays, with materials such as alginate and medium or heavy-bodied silicones. This reduces further the hydrostatic pressure and facilitates full seating of the tray.

Full seating

Regardless of the material used for the impression, it is imperative that special trays are not overloaded. You must ensure that they can be fully seated in order to achieve the required impression thickness, otherwise they fail to act as special trays, and they are probably no better than a good primary impression.

14 Compound and putty materials – handling and manipulation

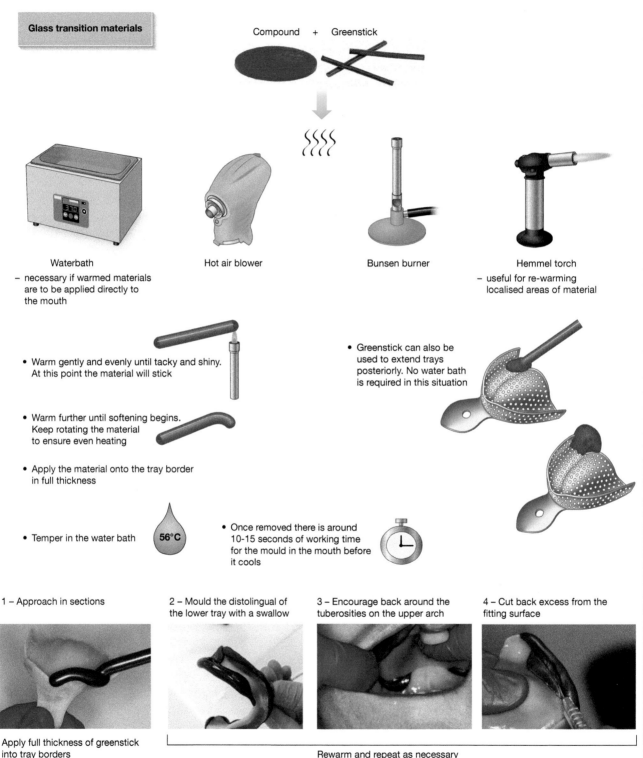

Figure 14.1 Compound materials – handling and manipulation

Glass transition materials

Compound + Greenstick

Waterbath
– necessary if warmed materials are to be applied directly to the mouth

Hot air blower

Bunsen burner

Hemmel torch
– useful for re-warming localised areas of material

- Warm gently and evenly until tacky and shiny. At this point the material will stick
- Warm further until softening begins. Keep rotating the material to ensure even heating
- Apply the material onto the tray border in full thickness
- Temper in the water bath 56°C
- Once removed there is around 10-15 seconds of working time for the mould in the mouth before it cools

- Greenstick can also be used to extend trays posteriorly. No water bath is required in this situation

1 – Approach in sections

Apply full thickness of greenstick into tray borders

2 – Mould the distolingual of the lower tray with a swallow

3 – Encourage back around the tuberosities on the upper arch

4 – Cut back excess from the fitting surface

Rewarm and repeat as necessary

Removable Prosthodontics at a Glance, First Edition. James Field and Claire Storey. © 2020 James Field and Claire Storey. Published 2020 by John Wiley & Sons Ltd.
Companion Website: www.wiley.com/go/field/removable

It is important that you understand the full range of materials at your disposal, their strengths and limitations, and how to employ them properly. Afford yourself the opportunity – both at dental school and thereafter – to play purposefully with a range of materials. Removable prosthodontics offers a unique opportunity in this respect, given that most procedures involving the manipulation of materials are non-invasive and reversible.

You will find that you are able to control some materials better than others. It may also be the case that specific situations dictate the material of choice. The remainder of this chapter considers important aspects of handling and manipulation of compound, greenstick and putty. Alginate is discussed in Chapter 11.

Compound and greenstick

These materials have a glass transition temperature of around 56 °C and so they need to be heated either with a flame, a hot air burner, or a water bath. On any occasion that you are moulding material in the mouth, you must ensure that it is tempered to no more than 60 °C. The most predictable way to do this is to use a water bath. If you are confident, you can also use running warm water. At the point when the water feels hot to touch, it is *usually* still a safe temperature in the mouth. If in doubt, take a sip of the running water from a cup to test it.

If the material is being used to form a tray extension, then the material will have cooled before using it in the patient's mouth; in this case a water bath is not needed.

When applying the material, the tray needs to be dry in order for the material to adhere effectively. At this point it can be reliably reheated and remoulded without it lifting from the tray. The ability to reheat and remould makes these materials an excellent choice for difficult cases. However, once a relatively thick amount of compound or greenstick has cooled, it takes a disproportionately long time to warm it up again – so bear this is mind when using large volumes.

Compound

Compound is most often available as 'cakes', either trapezoid or round in shape. If warming in water, try to sit the cake within an alginate mixing bowl to avoid the material sticking to the sink or the water bath walls. Once the material is unable to support itself, it is ready to apply to the tray. Compound is relatively viscous and so it will tend to easily displace the soft tissues and overextend sulci. However, it is excellent at supporting itself as it cools, and so it records distal aspects of anatomy like tuberosities and retromolar pads effectively. Unlike alginate or silicone, it will withstand distortion when the impression is poured up. Where large amounts are used across the arch, it is possible to rewarm localised areas with a hot air burner or a pin flame. Again, this should be tempered before re-seating in the mouth.

Greenstick

Greenstick has a bad name for itself because its use is rather technique-sensitive – but it is an incredibly useful and diagnostic material. Whilst it can be used for support in small edentulous areas, it is most useful for extending trays and border moulding. The sticks are purposefully designed with a particular thickness – and they are most effective when used in this way (Figure 14.1). As a border moulding material, it is important not to warm the material first in water – it should be warmed in air or a flame until it becomes shiny and tacky. Warm the material *slowly* until it starts to begin to flop (Figure 14.1). At this point it can be applied directly to the dry tray at its full thickness. It should then be tempered briefly before moulding in the mouth. There is no need for greenstick to be heated so much that it bubbles, like pizza cheese, or drips onto the bench. Once tempered, there is a window of around 10–15 seconds before it becomes too cool to mould effectively. Look for active material displacement, which will reassure you that the material is recording a functional sulcus. I often see greenstick being 'traced' onto the tray in small volumes. This is unproductive as the material cools too quickly and is never presented in sufficient volume to be moulded away from the functional sulcus. For border moulding complete arches, it is useful to approach sections of the arch in turn (Figure 14.1). Greenstick can be used to place a palatal stop, which reduces voids during the working impression. It is then helpful to record the buccal and labial sulcus on each side, then the tuberosities, and finally to communicate with a small addition of material across the post-dam. This final increment should sit *onto* the palatal aspect of the trimmed tray – not distal to it. Do not proceed to the wash impression until you are happy that the borders are moulded correctly. Trim excess material that has extended onto the fitting surface. If you are developing a border seal, a 'squelching' sensation indicates that the border seal is compromised, typically around the tuberosities or post-dam.

Difficult areas

An excellent method of ensuring full recording of the tuberosities and post-dam is to place greenstick into the fit surface of the tray and encourage excess material, which escapes distally, back up and against the required anatomy (Figure 14.1). If using alginate or silicone, it *is possible* to pre-load into this area with a syringe to help record them fully, but the material will quickly slump and flow away. On the lower arch, greenstick can also be placed into the tray over the pear-shaped and retromolar pads, and then excess can be encouraged back against the tray and into the disto-lingual sulcus (whilst also including border moulding with a swallow, and buccal moulding, to account for buccinator's attachment).

Putty

Clinical putty is available as a catalyst and base putty which need to be mixed together. The most efficient way to do this is on the bench top, akin to needing dough. This ensures a homogeneous mix and keeps the material cool, maximising your working time. The material provides a quicker alternative to warming and moulding compound – although it cannot be modified once it has set. Putty also needs to be encouraged back up to the anatomy around edentulous areas, because it has a tendency to drag. Adhesive should also be applied to the tray before using putty in large edentulous areas or free-end saddles. Putties and heavy-bodied silicones can also be used to carry out border moulding on trays – but again, the tray must be dry and adhesive must be applied beneath. Once the putty is placed onto the periphery, it is helpful to wet the border under the tap before moulding in the mouth. This results in a much more accurate and smooth border.

15 Recording an upper functional impression

Figure 15.1 Recording an upper functional impression

A systematic approach to border moulding

- Approach sections on the special tray in turn – typically the anterior segments first, then buccal, and then finally the tuberosities and the post dam

- Active tissue moulding by the clinician, with the patient relaxed

- Ask the patient to carry out exaggerated movements such as saying 'ooo' and 'eee'

- Record the restrictions of the coronoid process by asking the patient to move their jaw left and right

Most common faults

- Inadequate capturing of the tuberosities
- Overloaded trays
- Trays not being fully seated
- Inadequate border moulding

Tray extensions

- Buccal and labial
- Posterior

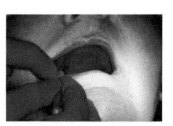

A watercolour pencil being used to trace the vibrating line intra orally

This can then be picked up on the special tray (image below) in order to help define the posterior border

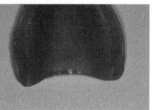

Border moulding

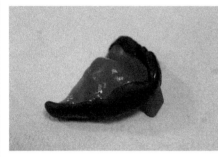

Buccal and labial

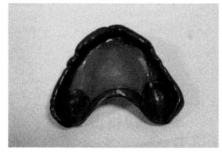

Tuberosities and post dam (encourage greenstick back up and around the tuberosities and across the post dam)

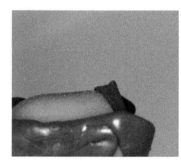

Creating your own post dam with greenstick

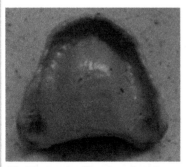

Wash impression (do not overload the tray, and ensure it is fully seated with plenty of functional moulding)

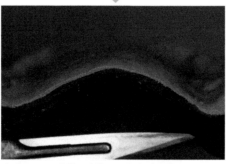

A clear prescription at the posterior border – note the even thickness of wash material

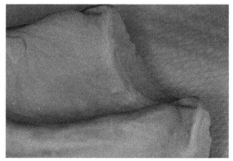

Scribing your own post dam on the master cast

Removable Prosthodontics at a Glance, First Edition. James Field and Claire Storey. © 2020 James Field and Claire Storey. Published 2020 by John Wiley & Sons Ltd.
Companion Website: www.wiley.com/go/field/removable

The vast majority of patients who are struggling to retain their upper dentures are suffering from significant denture over- or underextension. The stage at which the extensions are most easily and accurately recorded is during the functional (or working, major) impression. At this stage, effective tray extension and border moulding will dictate the limiting anatomy and result in a stable prosthesis. Making adjustments at a later stage is troublesome – not only in terms of identifying exactly *where* a denture is overextended – but by *how much*. In my opinion, time spent at this stage is time very well spent.

Checking the special tray

At this stage the tray must be checked for adaptation and extension. This can only reliably be achieved if tried in the patient's mouth. Trying trays on the casts, especially in the absence of tissue stops, can result in inappropriate tray alterations. The tray border should sit 2–3 mm clear of any limiting anatomy. It will act as a carrier so that the actual border anatomy can be recorded with a mouldable material such as greenstick, or during the wash impression. The posterior sulcal extensions can be assessed by holding the tray lightly in the mouth whilst reflecting the sulcus outwards and downwards. The patient needs to be relaxed, with the mouth 'half-closed', for this approach to be successful. If you can feel the tissues pulling the tray down, then it is still overextended. It is also possible to carry out a diagnostic 'wash' impression with light-bodied silicone, or alginate, which will show areas of over- or underextension. The posterior border can be marked intraorally using an indelible autoclavable pencil; if it is located correctly, when the patient's soft palate resonates during speech (typically saying 'ahhh') only the distal aspect of the line will move. Full posterior movement of the line indicates that it should be placed mesially. Once it is located correctly, seating the tray in the mouth should record any overextension onto the tray itself (which can be trimmed back) – or failing that, a tray deficit should be noticeable either directly or using a mirror.

Important functional anatomy

It is important to extend the impression into the *entire functional sulcus*. Flangeless or socket-fit complete dentures will not readily develop a border seal, and patients should be warned of this explicitly if they request or require such designs. The impression should also fully capture the *tuberosities* where necessary – not just in the horizontal plane, but extending up and around the hamular notch (Figure 15.1). Finally, the palate must be adequately captured, without voids, extending back to *the vibrating line*. This anatomical boundary is usually bordered on the distal aspect by the fovea palatini. Capturing this junction between the hard and soft palate for complete dentures means that a border seal can be maintained between the tuberosities. The special tray should be adjusted to meet these anatomical requirements.

Posterior border

Ideally, the posterior border of the denture should be clearly defined within the impression – either by a clear boundary on the impression itself (Figure 15.1) or by marking the vibrating line onto the impression. The related technical stage traditionally involves carving a 'cupid's bow' or 'post-dam' into the working cast, taking into account the degree of tissue compressibility across the posterior palatal arch. This creates an artificial 'peak' on the posterior denture border, which sits into the soft tissues and facilitates the maintenance of a border seal. If the posterior border is not defined, then the technician will assume its position, its contour and its depth. Some clinicians request their working cast to be returned so that they can carve the post-dam themselves. It is also possible, using a self-supporting material like greenstick, to create your own post-dam during the actual working impression (Figure 15.1). The advantage here is that you are able to make an immediate assessment about how stable and retentive the denture base is likely to be. Furthermore, the contour and depth of the post-dam are defined by the patient's *actual* anatomy.

It is quite possible to obtain all of the functional information in alginate, or silicone, in one go. However, I prefer, certainly in difficult cases, and when teaching this to students for the first time, to split this process into two stages.

Developing the peripheral extensions

This involves using greenstick or putty peripherally first, to ensure accurate functional border moulding. Areas of under- or overextension can be identified and rectified without the complications of a wash material. The degree of displacement and (for complete dentures) the border seal, can then be assessed prior to commencing the wash. See Chapter 14 for details on material behaviour and border moulding.

The wash impression

Adhesive should be applied to the tray when using silicone or alginate. It is critical *not to overload the tray* with material, otherwise it loses its function as a close-fitting special tray. Remind yourself of the spacing that you requested; loading a tray with zinc oxide eugenol, for example, is akin to icing a cake's surface, rather than 'filling up' the void within the tray. Ensure coverage of the full tray surface including up and over the tray extensions. For complete dentures, failing to cover the entire periphery often means that a border seal is achieved upon seating, but excess material is then unable to flow peripherally and escape. The impression should be seated slowly to avoid unnecessary hydrostatic pressure. Ensure that the tray is *fully and evenly seated and continue the border moulding* process in cycles until the material has set. Remind the patient to remain calm and relaxed during this stage to ensure adequate border moulding. Impressions should be removed by breaking the border seal around one of the tuberosities, rather than 'wiggling' the impression free. This approach is less likely to cause distortions. Working impressions for complete dentures should be rinsed and tried back in, in order to assess retention and stability.

Partial dentures

It is still important to ensure that partially dentate special trays are appropriately extended. This is still often forgotten with partial dentures. Free-end saddles should be treated with the same respect as for complete dentures. Overextension and displacement can still cause significant problems with partial dentures, more so if they are actively retained – in this case, overextension will often cause ulceration rather than displacement (or even both).

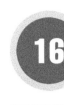

16 Recording a lower functional impression

Figure 16.1 Recording a lower functional impression

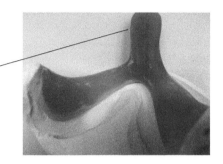

Tray extensions

- Upright handle to avoid displacing the tissues
- Reflect the labial sulcus and visually inspect (no sulcus means no tray extension!)
- Retract the buccal tissues
- Ask the patient to lift and protrude the tongue

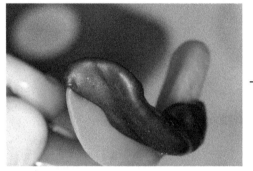

- Buccal and labial aspects should be recorded first – functional border moulding including 'ooo' and 'eee' sounds to account for modiolus

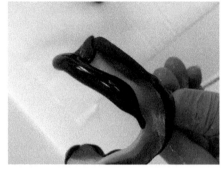

- Record the distolingual extensions with a swallow
- Record the lingual sulcus by pushing on the handle with the tongue and lifting the tongue

Partial functional impression

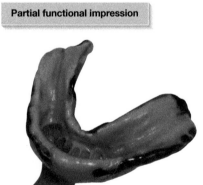

- The same principles apply for partial lower functional impressions, except you should use alginate or silicone for the wash impression

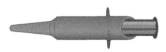

- An alginate syringe can help to deliver wash material distolingually and posteriorly but the alginate must be supported by the tray, or its extensions

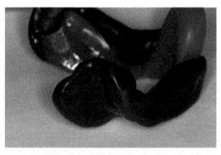

- Check stability in the mouth prior to a wash impression

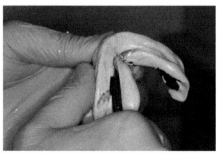

- If using Zinc Oxide Eugenol, fillet away ridge detail to prevent the denture base nipping the tissues

Removable Prosthodontics at a Glance, First Edition. James Field and Claire Storey. © 2020 James Field and Claire Storey. Published 2020 by John Wiley & Sons Ltd.
Companion Website: www.wiley.com/go/field/removable

The vast majority of patients who are struggling to retain their lower dentures are suffering from significant over- or underextension – but also placement of the lower anterior teeth outside the neutral zone. The latter is discussed further in Chapter 24.

Checking the special tray

As discussed in the previous chapter, the tray border should sit 2–3 mm clear of any limiting anatomy. The anterior and posterior sulcal extensions can be assessed by holding the tray lightly in the mouth whilst reflecting the sulcus outwards and upwards. The patient needs to be relaxed, with the mouth 'half-closed', for this approach to be successful. Unlike the upper arch, it is much easier to see tray extensions directly on the lower. If the tray reaches the full depth of the functional sulcus then it must be trimmed back. If you can feel the tissues pulling the tray up, then it is still overextended. The patient should also be asked to raise the tongue to the roof of the mouth, and to protrude it laterally and anteriorly. It also useful for the patient to push against the anterior tray handle with their tongue, which activates genioglossus. Swallowing will activate palatoglossus, although this is quite difficult to carry out without stabilising the tray – as a result, tray displacements are missed. It is better to ask the patient to swallow when you are ready to record border movements actively. Finally, it is also possible to carry out a diagnostic 'wash' impression with light-bodied silicone, or alginate, which will show areas of over- or underextension.

Important functional anatomy

On lower arch arches presenting with free-end saddles, the impression should fully capture the *pear-shaped pads* (which represent the scar tissue from the last standing molar) and partially cover the *retromolar pads*. It is also important to account for the insertion of the buccinator into the retromolar pad and the confluence of modiolus. These anatomical features are discussed further in Chapter 10. The special tray should be adjusted to meet these anatomical requirements.

Labial sulcus

With severely atrophic lower ridges, it is common for stock trays to exaggerate the labial sulcus. Without due attention, this then results in special trays which are also overextended. Special attention should be paid to the tray extension in this area. Do not be afraid to adjust the tray until it is stable in function. No sulcus means there should be no tray extension. The tray handle may restrict border moulding in this area and you may feel that you also need to trim this back to facilitate the process.

Posterior and disto-lingual anatomy

The antero-posterior and rotational stability of a denture sitting on a severely atrophic ridge will be largely determined by the distal and disto-lingual extensions. If your special tray happens to fall short of the retromolar pad, then it must be extended adequately prior to the wash impression. The posterior and disto-lingual anatomy is particularly tricky to record properly and

there are advantages to spending some time developing the posterior extensions prior to taking a wash impression.

Developing the peripheral extensions

This involves using greenstick or putty peripherally first, to ensure accurate functional border moulding. The material should be applied to sections of the tray in turn, and the border moulding procedures repeated each time. These can be based on soft tissue manipulation, patient movements, or both. On the lower there may be a need for more patient involvement because of the presence of the tongue. It can be helpful to ask patients to say 'oooo' and 'eeee'. Most of the time there is little point border moulding the periphery buccal to any standing teeth – the denture will not be extended into this area. However, it is equally as important to ensure that trays are not *over*extended in this area, otherwise they can affect the seating of the tray and its relationship to the denture-bearing area elsewhere in the arch.

When reaching the posterior aspect, it is useful to place a small amount of border moulding material onto the pear-shaped and retromolar area. When the tray is seated and the excess material escapes peripherally, this should be encouraged back up against the tray in order to begin to record finer muscle attachments and subtly engage undercuts lingual to the ridge. The same movements that were used to check the tray should be repeated in order to record the functional border.

It is much less common to achieve a border seal in the lower arch, although this is possible with careful adaptation to the pear-shaped and retromolar pads, and the disto-lingual sulcus.

The wash impression

Adhesive should be applied to the tray when using silicone or alginate. Overloading of the tray tends to be less critical on the lower edentulous ridge, but can still be a problem with multiple bounded saddles. Once again, the impression should be seated slowly to avoid unnecessary hydrostatic pressure. Ensure that the tray is *fully and evenly seated* and *continue the border moulding* process in cycles until the material has set. This includes raising the tongue to the roof of the mouth, and protruding it laterally and anteriorly. Also ask the patient to push against the anterior tray handle with their tongue and to half-close to *encourage a swallow*. Remind the patient to remain calm and relaxed during this stage to ensure adequate border moulding. Working impressions for complete dentures should be rinsed and tried back in, in order to assess stability. Often, atrophic lower edentulous ridges present with a thin fin of tissue along the crest of the ridge. It can be useful to dissect this away with a scalpel in order to prevent the denture 'nipping' (Figure 16.1). This technique will be discussed further later.

Partial dentures

Elastic impression materials are required for partial dentures (silicone or alginate). Do not forget that free-end saddles should be treated with the same respect as for complete dentures – overextension and displacement can still cause significant problems. An alginate syringe can be a useful adjunct for delivering alginate disto-lingually, but do not forget that if the alginate is not supported by the tray, then it is likely to distort when the impression is poured up.

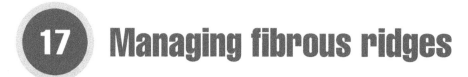

17 Managing fibrous ridges

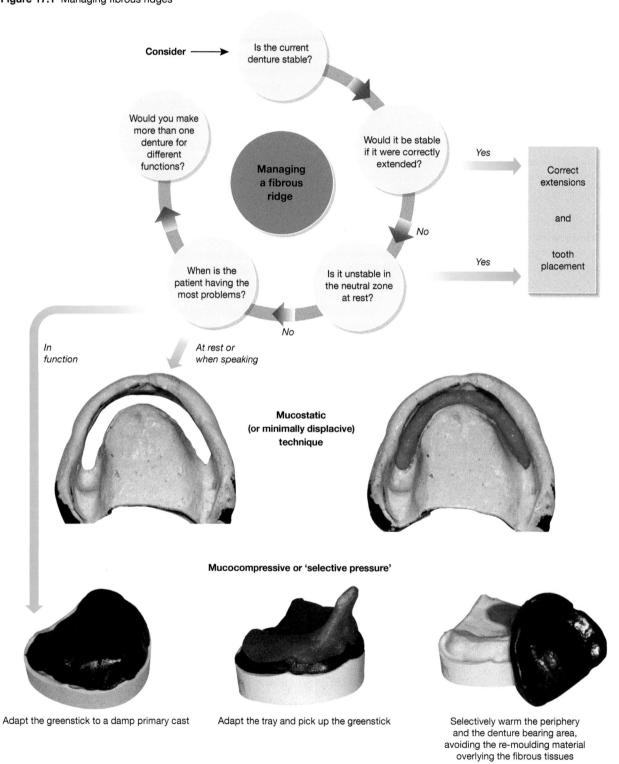

Figure 17.1 Managing fibrous ridges

Consider → Is the current denture stable?

Would it be stable if it were correctly extended? — *Yes* → Correct extensions and tooth placement

Is it unstable in the neutral zone at rest? — *Yes*

Managing a fibrous ridge

Would you make more than one denture for different functions?

When is the patient having the most problems?

No

No

In function

At rest or when speaking

Mucostatic (or minimally displacive) technique

Mucocompressive or 'selective pressure'

Adapt the greenstick to a damp primary cast

Adapt the tray and pick up the greenstick

Selectively warm the periphery and the denture bearing area, avoiding the re-moulding material overlying the fibrous tissues

Removable Prosthodontics at a Glance, First Edition. James Field and Claire Storey. © 2020 James Field and Claire Storey. Published 2020 by John Wiley & Sons Ltd.
Companion Website: www.wiley.com/go/field/removable

Occasionally you may notice that edentulous ridges are mobile, or 'fibrous'. This is most common in the upper anterior region, the tuberosities and the lower retromolar region. Occasionally it can affect the arch more generally. Whilst there is little evidence for the cause, upper anterior fibrous ridges are often attributed to the combination of lower natural anterior teeth, opposing the upper edentulous ridge. You may hear the term 'flabby' ridge – although we tend not to use this term in front of patients, because it can seem rather discourteous in the absence of any other explanation!

Fibrous ridges are nothing to be worried about – but they do have the potential to cause denture instability. During the denture assessment it is important to investigate the boundaries of the mobile tissue – and in which directions it appears to displace when loaded. It is also important to bring this relevant anatomy to your patient's attention and describe the potential problems that they may encounter – even if they are not currently reporting any issues. If the patient has a current denture, then make sure that you spend some time assessing its fit and its stability, so that you can appreciate how much of an impact the fibrous tissue might have. Whilst fibrous ridges might impact on denture stability, they should not really affect the degree of retention. Sometimes it is useful to reassure patients that although they might feel the denture moving slightly in function, if well made, it will not displace from the denture-bearing area.

So what can be done to try to minimise the effects of the mobile tissue? Whilst for severe cases, localised surgery may provide an effective solution, most of the time we can cater for the mobile tissue within our working impression. It is, however, important to understand the following:

• *Is the current denture stable?* – If the current denture is stable at rest and in function, then there is little need to be concerned about the fibrous tissue during denture construction
• *If not, is the instability because of poor extensions?* – When patients have a fibrous ridge, it is common to attribute denture instability to the fibrous ridge itself. Make sure that the problem is not compounded by over- or underextension into the sulci, or across the denture-bearing area. This will allow you to make a more informed judgement about the likely impact of the fibrous tissue
• *Is the denture sitting outside the neutral zone at rest?* – The neutral zone will be considered in Chapter 24, but whether the denture's polished surfaces are correctly placed or not will impact on denture stability, similar to considering the extensions. Ensure that this is not compounding the problem.

Ultimately, if the fibrous ridge *is* affecting denture stability, then it is equally as important to understand *when your patient is having the most problems*. This key question should allow you to determine which approach will be most effective in managing the fibrous ridge. If the patient is having difficulty at rest or during speech, then the tissue is likely recoiling against the denture base and causing displacement. In this case, the area of fibrous tissue should be respected and recorded mucostatically (Figure 17.1). If the patient is having most problems during mastication, then the tissue is allowing itself to be compressed during function and causing displacement. In this case, the area of fibrous tissue should be compressed during the working impression (Figure 17.1).

Clearly there are situations where the patient would benefit from both a mucostatic and a mucocompressed tissue – and so communication with the patient is very important. The patient should understand that it may not be possible to create a conventional denture that is stable all of the time. In some rare cases we have made patients two or even three dentures for use at different times – exact replicas, apart from the way in which they interact with the fibrous tissue. We will now consider techniques to record tissue mucostatically and mucocompressively.

Mucostatic

Mucostatic impressions are sometimes referred to as 'minimally displacive' – it must be understood that it is quite hard to construct a denture that will not load the fibrous tissue *at all*. In this case, we should use materials for our primary impression that minimally distort the fibrous tissue, such as alginate or silicone, rather than compound or putty. This will mean that the special tray is already somewhat respectful of the tissue's normal resting anatomy. The technique requires the use of a 'window' within the working impression tray to allow the tissue to be recorded without being compressed. It is possible to ask the laboratory to pre-cut a window into the tray – and in order for this to be accurate, you must communicate (either by drawing on the primary impression or drawing a diagram) where the window should be. The impression is developed as normal and after taking the wash impression, material is cut away from the window and the impression is re-seated. A mucostatic material such as light-bodied silicone is then introduced around the fibrous tissue to restore the impression (Figure 17.1). If using a two-stage technique, and first establishing the border extensions, it is useful to cut the window yourself *after* you have finished the peripheral border moulding; otherwise the window will prevent you from establishing a border seal.

Mucocompressive

Many classic texts consider a 'selective pressure' technique. Here, a primary impression is taken in a mucocompressive material such as compound. The special tray is then adapted with greenstick against the primary cast. Ensure that the cast is soaked first to prevent the greenstick adhering. After cooling, the technique then requires the greenstick to be heated and moulded selectively in all but the fibrous areas. The borders are then moulded normally, with or without a wash impression. In reality, this is a *very* technique-sensitive method. In my experience it is sufficient to record a primary impression in a mucocompressive material (compound) and then request a special tray to be constructed with no perforations and no spacer over the fibrous area. A relatively mucocompressive material should then be used for the wash impression. In this case, zinc oxide eugenol will behave mucocompressively because of the lack of spacer.

In any case, requesting a permanent base for the jaw relation stage means that you can judge the outcome of your chosen technique sooner, and ensure a more accurate prescription.

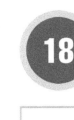

18 Denture bases

Figure 18.1 Denture bases

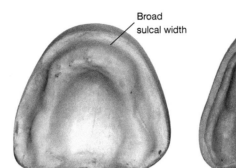
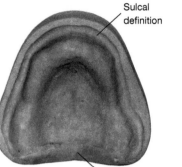

Broad sulcal width

Sulcal definition

Primary cast (left) in comparison to a working cast (right) for a complete denture – note the differences in sulcal width, depth and definition

Minimal posterior anatomy

Posterior definition

Advantages of a permanent base

- Able to definitively check comfort, stability and retention
- Able to make definitive permanent changes
- More stability and accuracy when recording jaw relations
- Able to remove wax down to the base without distortion or collapse

Advantages of a temporary base

- Avoids the problem of heel clash
- Able to scribe your own post-dam on the master cast
- Greater flexibility when inter-arch space is limited

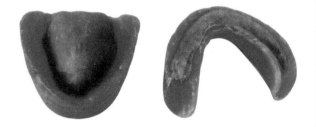

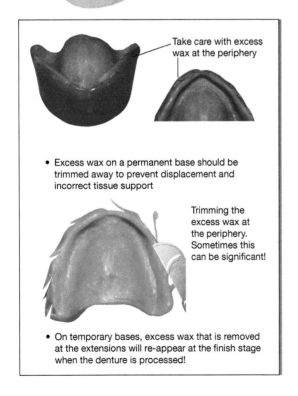

Take care with excess wax at the periphery

- Excess wax on a permanent base should be trimmed away to prevent displacement and incorrect tissue support

Trimming the excess wax at the periphery. Sometimes this can be significant!

- On temporary bases, excess wax that is removed at the extensions will re-appear at the finish stage when the denture is processed!

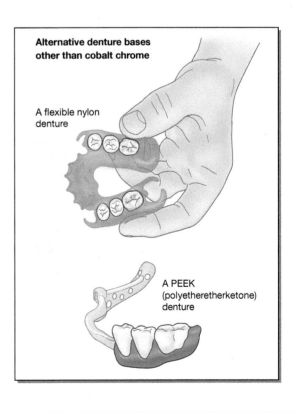

Alternative denture bases other than cobalt chrome

A flexible nylon denture

A PEEK (polyetheretherketone) denture

Removable Prosthodontics at a Glance, First Edition. James Field and Claire Storey. © 2020 James Field and Claire Storey. Published 2020 by John Wiley & Sons Ltd.
Companion Website: www.wiley.com/go/field/removable

The finished fitting surface of your prosthesis will be derived from your master (or working) impression. Although it is possible in some cases to obtain a very detailed and functional impression with a well-adjusted stock tray, it should normally be the case that the degree of functional anatomy recorded for the master cast is significantly more detailed than that recorded for the primary (Figure 18.1; note the differences in sulcal definition, depth and width). This discrepancy becomes significant if you are in the habit of requesting record blocks alongside your special trays; in the interests of time, we often see registration stages and major impressions being carried out at the same appointment. The problem here is that the record blocks, which have been constructed on the primary casts, are then seated onto the working casts in order to articulate the models. Most laboratory technicians will tell you that they dislike this approach, because they find it almost impossible to accurately seat the blocks. In the interests of accuracy and longer term expedience, I would recommend using registration blocks constructed on working casts. For cobalt chrome partial dentures, this is never really a concern, because the working impression must be taken first in order for the framework to be waxed-up and cast. Once it has been tried in, the metal framework will then have wax record blocks attached to its edentulous areas ready for the registration process.

Types of denture base

For partial denture construction it is most convenient to proceed through the registration and try-in stages using temporary denture bases. However, for complete dentures you can consider requesting that the record blocks are constructed on permanent bases. The merits of each approach are discussed below.

Permanent acrylic bases

In this case, the record blocks are constructed on the *actual* finished denture bases. It is common for the working cast to break or fracture during unflasking because of the rigid nature of the acrylic – and so expect to see defects on the returned working cast. Now that the base has been processed, the remaining cast is of little consequence, other than it is used to reliably and stably seat the block for articulation purposes.

Advantages of using permanent complete denture bases include:
• Provide a more stable block and therefore a more accurate recording of the jaw relationship
• Offer an opportunity to check definitively the comfort, adaptation, stability and retention of your finished denture base prior to fit
• Permit the removal of wax completely without the risk of the block collapsing
• Permanent base changes are retained throughout the remainder of the construction process
• You have less need to protect your working casts as they accompany the laboratory work back and forth

It is always worth checking how wax has been added to the denture base – the lip support should be derived from the crowns of the teeth only. Extending large volumes of wax up to the denture border is unnecessary and will undoubtedly compromise the sulcal adaptation and border seal. This excess wax should be trimmed away prior to the bases being placed into the mouth (Figure 18.1). This is much easier to manage with a permanent acrylic base beneath the wax. On occasions it may also be necessary to augment or further extend the denture base – and this might happen if you notice a discrepancy or an underextension. Permanent bases are relatively easy to augment using compound or greenstick, without the base perishing. Temporary bases are notoriously difficult, if not impossible, to extend reliably. In any case, if a modification to the base was needed, a final wash impression to pick up the fine detail would be saved until the dentures had been tried in and were found to be satisfactory. At this point, any undercuts should be removed from the fitting surface and a wash impression taken using a closed mouth technique (with the patient closing into their intercuspal position against the opposing arch). When utilising permanent bases for registration and try-in stages, it may be necessary to ask the patient to remove their old denture half an hour or so before the appointment to allow the tissues to recoil. If you know that you made a retentive impression but at first insertion the permanent base seems to have lost retention, do not panic. Be patient, calm and reassuring before moving on to troubleshoot other factors.

Temporary bases

Temporary bases can be formed entirely from wax, sometimes reinforced with a stainless-steel arch wire. This is quite typical for partial registration blocks. Alternatively, the temporary base may be constructed from shellac or light-cured acrylic, with wax rims attached. In any case, it is often when we are adjusting *temporary* bases that distortions occur. If you need to alter a record block on a temporary base, be sure to firstly place it back onto the working cast, so that it can be supported whilst you modify it.

Advantages of using temporary complete denture bases include:
• The possible avoidance, or facilitation of the management, of heel clash during registration
• The ability to scribe your own post-dam onto the master cast at the chair side before the base is definitively processed
• Greater flexibility when interarch space is limited

The main drawbacks of temporary bases include compromised retention and the inability to modify the base definitively without going back a stage and taking a new working impression.

Alternative denture base materials

Alternatives to acrylic resin and cobalt chrome seem to come and go – and we will see more of these innovations with further developments in 3D printing and laser sintering. Flexible dentures made from Nylon have been available for some time – although for partial dentures we should exercise caution. This is primarily because a flexible denture base fails to gain support from across the full arch from the hard and soft tissues. By its very nature, it flexes – which means that it can be loaded differentially and even place excessive torqueing forces onto abutment teeth. Rests and clasps do not behave in the same way and yet we use traditional cobalt chrome design principles to construct frameworks. Polyetheretherketone and polyketoneketone bases show a degree of promise although they are still up to 10 times more flexible than cobalt chrome and cannot be utilised in thin section. At the time of writing, I advise caution with these materials until further clinical evidence of their effectiveness and support for oral health is available.

19 Recording the maxillo-mandibular relationship

Figure 19.1 Recording the maxilla-mandibular relationship

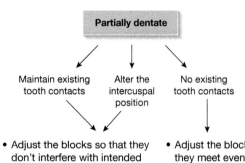

Partially dentate

Maintain existing tooth contacts → Alter the intercuspal position → No existing tooth contacts

- Adjust the blocks so that they don't interfere with intended tooth contacts

- Adjust the blocks so that they meet evenly at the required vertical dimension. Where possible, cut notches in the record blocks that oppose natural teeth

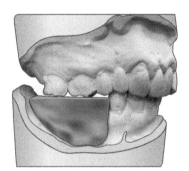

- Adjust the blocks so that they don't interfere with intended tooth contacts

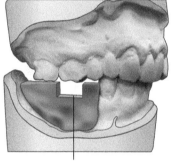

- Cut deep opposing notches

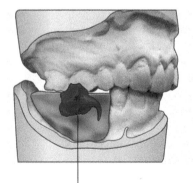

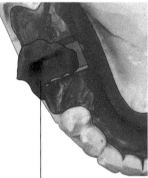

- Register passively with silicone paste

Edentulous

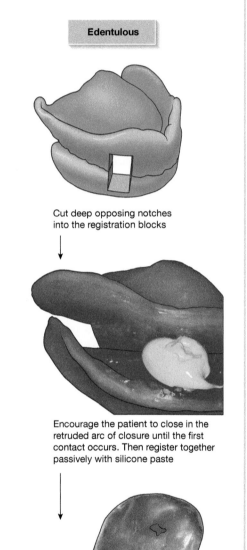

Cut deep opposing notches into the registration blocks

Encourage the patient to close in the retruded arc of closure until the first contact occurs. Then register together passively with silicone paste

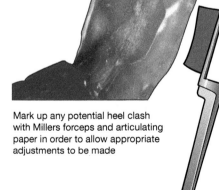

Mark up any potential heel clash with Millers forceps and articulating paper in order to allow appropriate adjustments to be made

Millers forceps

Removable Prosthodontics at a Glance, First Edition. James Field and Claire Storey. © 2020 James Field and Claire Storey. Published 2020 by John Wiley & Sons Ltd.
Companion Website: www.wiley.com/go/field/removable

The term 'registration' is often used to encompass both *the recording of the relationship between the upper and the lower arches* and *the prescription for the placement of the denture teeth.* In fact, these are two very different processes, which should be carried out independently of one another. Placement of the upper and lower teeth is considered in Chapters 20–22 respectively. The remainder of this chapter will consider the fundamental aspects of actually *recording* the relationship between the upper and lower blocks.

The denture bases

The merits of employing a permanent denture base for the registration stage of complete dentures were discussed in Chapter 18. The more stable the registration base, the more accurate and reliable the registration process is going to be. This is also an opportunity to make any necessary changes to the denture base in order to improve the comfort, fit or the extensions. Changes made to temporary bases will be lost, unless a new working impression is taken. Partial denture registration blocks are almost always provided as temporary bases. You may find that it is useful to employ some denture adhesive in order to stabilise the bases if you have problems with retention.

Natural tooth contacts in partially dentate patients

At this stage, the occlusal vertical dimension should have also been prescribed, and this is discussed further in Chapter 23. However, it is important to reinforce that for partially dentate patients, if you are working to existing tooth contacts, then it makes the process of recording the relationship between the upper and lower dentition simpler – and much easier to verify. Each block should be adjusted independently in the mouth to ensure that the natural contact(s) are maintained. Record blocks should act as *carriers* for a more accurate registration medium like silicone; patients should *not* be *biting* into wax with their natural teeth. The only noticeable contact should be between the natural teeth. The patient should be relaxed and the process should be passive. This will ensure that you obtain accurate and reproducible results. The process of accurately recording the relationship is described below.

The registration material

As mentioned earlier, the registration blocks should act as 'carriers' for a registration medium, such as a silicone paste. By cutting deep and retentive notches into the registration blocks, the paste can be introduced passively into the void, and record the detail of the opposing surface(s). This arrangement should then be disassembled for disinfection, and readily reassembled. It is a good idea to test the disassembly and reassembly before disinfection, and before the patient has left the chair, in case you find that it cannot be relocated easily – and should therefore be repeated. There is no need to create a thin layer of registration paste around the entire arch – this will interfere with the interocclusal relationship and can promote a slide. Instead, three or four points around the arch should be chosen, ensuring that the casts have at least tripod stability when reassembled, reducing the risk of rocking. One limitation of silicone which should be noted is that it often picks up *more* detail on an opposing natural dentition than is replicated by an alginate impression and as

such, the registration matrices have a tendency to 'bounce' when the casts are mounted together. To overcome this, the fine fissures recorded in the silicone registration matrices can be sliced away with a scalpel. It is also possible to smudge carding wax into the occlusal fissures of the natural teeth prior to taking the registration. In this way, the fine detail is not replicated in the silicone – only the cusp tips are important here.

It is not reliable to heat or roughen the occlusal wax and ask the patient to 'bite' together. This results in a relationship that is often irreproducible. Furthermore, warming the wax surface can alter the occlusal relationship and distort the prescription for where the technician should place the teeth.

A passive process

The more passive the registration process, the more accurate the result. Patients should be completely relaxed and reclined to around 45 degrees. Encourage your patient to relax their shoulders by applying some light pressure on them, and ask them to feel their jaw dropping backwards as they relax. Try this yourself – close in and out of intercuspal position whilst looking forwards – and then slowly tilt your head backwards. Feel your jaw retruding, and slowly close – the majority of people who are dentate will feel an early contact in the retruded arc of closure. Whilst we often use bi-manual manipulation to encourage patients into this arc, *often* this really is not necessary and can, in fact, cause inaccuracies. If you take the time to explain what you want to achieve, patients can actually be extremely helpful in obtaining an accurate registration. The problem is that many dentists refer to this process as a 'bite' stage, which gives the patient the wrong idea about what they should be doing. Patients should slowly close until they feel *something* touch – and then stop. That might be the intended contact(s) – but it might also be an aberrant contact or heel clash of the denture bases. This can be an extremely diagnostic process if your patient is understanding and cooperative.

The process

When you are ready, and the patient is clear about the process, prepare the registration paste. Seat the block(s) and slowly encourage your patient to passively close until they feel contact. Check this is reproducible and in the intended position. Upon contact with the block(s), syringe the registration paste into the voids in the blocks so that it records the opposing surface. Record all sections concurrently. It is important to manage the patient's mandibular position during the setting time – do not leave the patient to attend to other matters.

Checking the registration

Apart from being able to disassemble and reconstruct the registration, you should also inspect the relationship of the bases for heel clash – between bases if they are opposing – or heel clash on the master casts. The latter can usually be adjusted, but heel clash between a denture base should be corrected (usually by adjusting the base or increasing the occlusal vertical dimension) and re-recorded. If you suspect heel clash, either insert some GHM articulating paper between the bases and ask the patient to close or carry out the same procedure with a small amount of registration or pressure relief paste. Contact of the bases will be visible and can then be adjusted (Figure 19.1).

20 Prescribing the upper wax contour

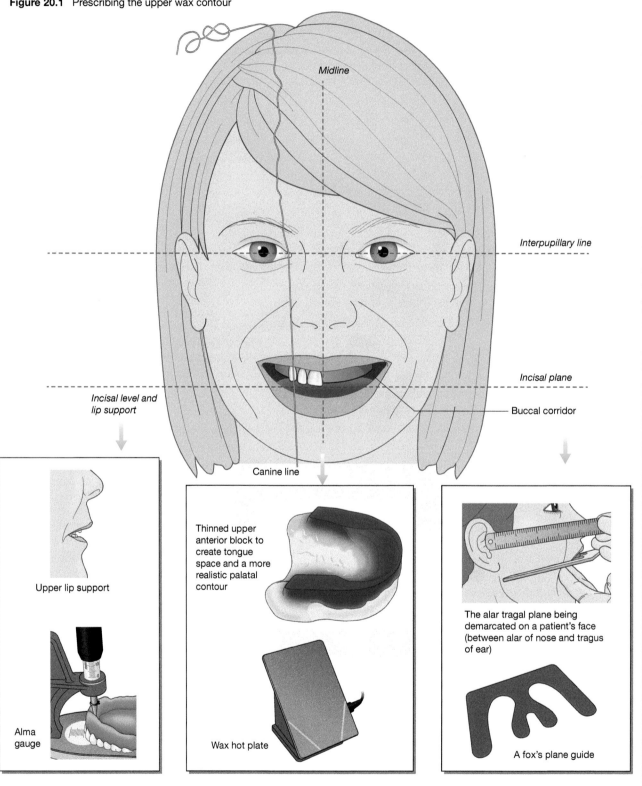

Figure 20.1 Prescribing the upper wax contour

Midline

Interpupillary line

Incisal plane

Buccal corridor

Incisal level and lip support

Canine line

Upper lip support

Alma gauge

Thinned upper anterior block to create tongue space and a more realistic palatal contour

Wax hot plate

The alar tragal plane being demarcated on a patient's face (between alar of nose and tragus of ear)

A fox's plane guide

Removable Prosthodontics at a Glance, First Edition. James Field and Claire Storey. © 2020 James Field and Claire Storey. Published 2020 by John Wiley & Sons Ltd.
Companion Website: www.wiley.com/go/field/removable

At this stage it is very important to revisit the treatment plan that you originally devised. Unless the presence of natural teeth dictates your prosthetic tooth positions, you have a degree of artistic licence; you should clearly note the specific aesthetic and occlusal features that you wish to prescribe. It is imperative that the registration block is tried in, and is comfortable and stable, prior to proceeding with this clinical stage. All modifications to the block should be made with care and precision. Rough wax work will make it hard for the technician to read your prescription – and it will also affect the relationship with the upper lip. Often at try-in dentists find that they seem to have prescribed an incisal level that is too high (resulting in inadequate exposure of the incisors). This is often because the lip rests further down on the refined waxwork and smooth denture teeth than it did on the rough block.

There are several features that should be prescribed on the upper block, and these are shown in Figure 20.1 and described below. As a rule of thumb, it is usually a good idea to *prescribe the upper tooth positions based on aesthetics.*

Using the previous denture as a guide

An Alma gauge is an invaluable piece of equipment that can save a lot of chairside time. The gauge allows you, using the incisive papilla as a consistent landmark, to measure the amount of lip support (horizontal reading) and the incisal level (vertical reading) provided by an upper denture. It is possible to use the existing denture's measurement to help inform your decision at the prescription stage and also to inform the technician how much lip support and what incisal level you would like on your registration block. This can save a lot of clinical time which is otherwise spent adding or removing wax and is discussed further in Chapter 27.

Lip support

Pay close attention to the wax rim and ensure that wax does not extend right up to the denture border. This is unnecessary – it will compromise your border seal (for complete dentures) and will provide an incorrect soft tissue support for the upper lip, resulting in a rolled appearance of the infranasal tissues. This can also happen if the denture base extensions are too thick. If this is the case, a permanent base can be adjusted before proceeding. Be careful with a temporary base, because these adjustments will be lost prior to processing, and will result in an altered lip support at the fit stage. The lip support should be derived from the crowns of the teeth only – and it is useful to remember this if you find yourself adding more wax, or indeed, taking it away. Only a strip of wax, around 1 cm high, needs to be added to or removed from the incisal aspect of the block. Patients can usually articulate whether they feel they would like the degree of lip support to be changed – and normally we would expect the angle formed between the upper lip and the base of the nose to be around 90 degrees – this is usually a good starting point (Figure 20.1). However, it is always worth reminding the patient that there is a sensitive interplay between aesthetics, stability and speech. Increasing the lip support significantly may result in a denture that is unstable in function, as it loses a direct relationship to the upper edentulous ridge upon which is should gain support.

Incisal level and the alar–tragal plane

A fox's plane guide can be used to assess the incisal plane and the alar–tragal plane (with which the occlusal surface should be parallel). It might seem straightforward to prescribe an incisal plane, but sometimes asymmetrical facial anatomy can make this challenging. Most often we tend to prescribe the incisal plane parallel to the interpupillary line. However, the lips themselves, the nose or even the ears can be used as reference points. If in doubt, assess which plane the existing denture incisors are parallel to and take it from there. It is easiest to adjust the block using a hot plate, which provides a flat surface. The amount of incisor showing changes with age and typically we would expect the incisor tips to contact the lower lip during labiodental fricatives (such as 'F').

It is a good idea to check the alar–tragal plane (the antero-posterior plane) early on in the process so that you already have an appreciation of how you might need to alter the wax block. For example, if you are about to raise the incisal level, it would be useful to know if you also need to remove wax anteriorly in order to correct the alar–tragal plane. The two can then be altered concurrently. Without this consideration, you may have to remove wax along the entire block, only to need to replace it again in one specific area. Adding wax in this way is much more difficult to achieve than levelling the occlusal plane with a hot plate. If in doubt, simply correct the occlusal plane first, and then address the incisal level. At least with this approach you are removing or adding wax across the entire block in an equal thickness.

Buccal corridors

Prescribing buccal corridors is often forgotten – and as a consequence the upper teeth can sometimes look falsely 'full' in the mouth. Whilst the upper block should prescribe teeth that sit over the edentulous ridge in order to maximise stability, upper teeth do not naturally contact the buccal mucosa in function. Ask someone to give you a big cheesy smile and you will notice a void between the buccal surfaces of the teeth and the buccal mucosa – these are known as buccal corridors. Failing to respect them can lead to speech problems and cheek biting. As a rule of thumb, prescribe the teeth over the edentulous ridge; at this point, if buccal corridors are missing, then hold the block obliquely onto the hot plate and bevel the edge of the block. This will tuck the buccal surfaces in medially and begin to allocate some buccal space.

Other useful markers

Once you have finishing making changes to your planes of reference, it is important to clearly mark the midline and the high smile line with a wax knife. It is also useful to mark the intended canine positions, but this is discussed further in Chapter 22.

Tongue space and assessing speech

Once you have prescribed your lip support, it is useful to pare out the palatal aspect of the block to replicate the expected tooth contour (Figure 20.1). A 1 cm thick wax rim will severely restrict the tongue, causing displacement, and makes assessment of speech very difficult.

21 Prescribing the lower wax contour

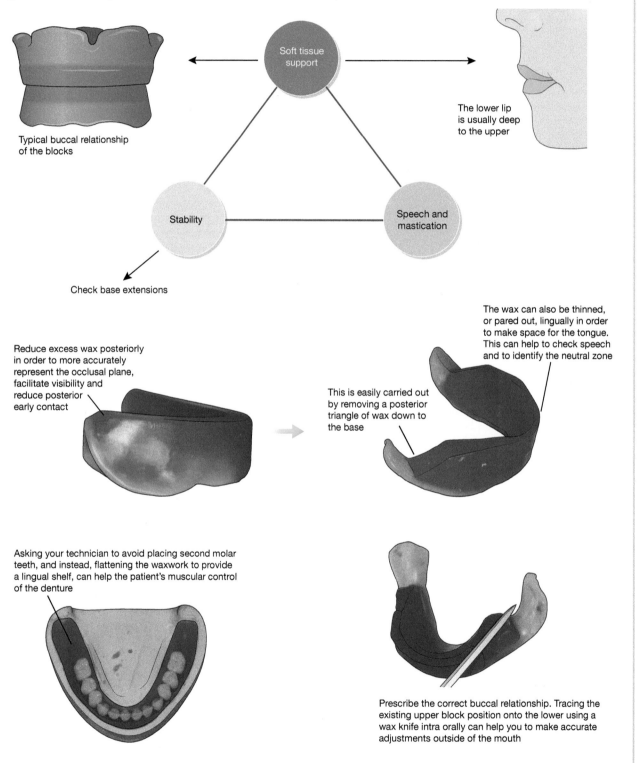

Figure 21.1 Prescribing the lower wax contour

Typical buccal relationship of the blocks

Soft tissue support

The lower lip is usually deep to the upper

Stability

Speech and mastication

Check base extensions

Reduce excess wax posteriorly in order to more accurately represent the occlusal plane, facilitate visibility and reduce posterior early contact

This is easily carried out by removing a posterior triangle of wax down to the base

The wax can also be thinned, or pared out, lingually in order to make space for the tongue. This can help to check speech and to identify the neutral zone

Asking your technician to avoid placing second molar teeth, and instead, flattening the waxwork to provide a lingual shelf, can help the patient's muscular control of the denture

Prescribe the correct buccal relationship. Tracing the existing upper block position onto the lower using a wax knife intra orally can help you to make accurate adjustments outside of the mouth

Removable Prosthodontics at a Glance, First Edition. James Field and Claire Storey. © 2020 James Field and Claire Storey. Published 2020 by John Wiley & Sons Ltd.
Companion Website: www.wiley.com/go/field/removable

The previous chapter described how the upper block should be primarily prescribed based on aesthetics and facial support – but a depleted lower dentition, or an edentulous arch, will often dictate that *stability* and *zones of neutrality* are the main drivers for prescription of the lower block. Once again, the patient should be reminded at this stage of the interplay between soft tissue support, stability and speech. It is therefore particularly important on the lower arch, especially labially, to check for base overextension prior to proceeding with the prescription. When standing in front of the patient, the labial tissues can be fully reflected to inspect the extensions directly.

It is common for lower complete registration blocks to be fabricated with discrepant occlusal planes; typically too high posteriorly, because the most superior aspect of the distal base extension is used as a reference. More often than not this plane is incorrect, and so removing the posterior triangle of wax can help – this keeps the posterior aspect, and its relationship to the upper block, visible. It also increases the efficiency of modification to the block.

For complete dentures it is worth considering the use of permanent bases – not only to ensure maximum stability – but also in case there is a need to permanently alter the bases to correct overextension, heel clash, or to remove segments of wax to execute a neutral zone impression (described in Chapter 22). If you are intending to carry out a neutral zone impression at the registration stage, then wax rims which are already missing the lower anterior portion can be requested. These are known as 'Manchester' rims – whilst they might seem easier to adjust, be careful not to fall into the habit of using these without prescribing the lower anterior tooth position. For partially dentate arches, especially on the lower anterior sextant, you may find that small saddle areas distort or detach easily from the main block. Do not worry too much about this – the adjacent teeth will give information about intended tooth positions, and it is unlikely that small bounded saddles will help with the accuracy of recording jaw relations. Similar to the upper arch, the presence of natural lower teeth might dictate your prescription in terms of arch-form and occlusal plane. With natural anterior lower teeth that are opposing an upper edentulous ridge, it is often important to revisit the upper block and pare out the wax palatally in order to accommodate the lower anteriors (prescribing an overbite). This is necessary in order to allow an appropriate occlusal vertical dimension and incisor relationship to be accounted for simultaneously.

The tongue

Aside from sulcular extensions and the neutral zone, the other factor that will impact significantly on lower denture stability is the tongue. This is made significantly more troublesome for patients who are not in the habit of wearing an existing lower prosthesis. As a muscle, the tongue can lose tone and become particularly unruly when allowed to passively occupy extra space. When prescribing the positions of the lower teeth, especially for complete dentures, it pays dividends to be mindful of how the tongue can be re-trained to help control the lower prosthesis. This requires a degree of perseverance by the patient – but also consider flattening the lingual aspect of the waxwork distally in order to provide a shelf upon which the tongue can rest and help to stabilise the denture. Also consider leaving off the lower second molars, which further increases the space available for the tongue to help stabilise the denture base.

Lip support

Once again, only a strip of wax, around 1 cm high, needs to be added to or removed from the incisal aspect of the block. In a class I skeletal base we would normally expect the lower lip to sit deep to the upper lip (Figure 21.1). Paying close attention to the stability of the lower block in an antero-posterior direction may mean you need to reduce the lip support significantly in order to account for the activity of the lower lip and mentalis muscles.

Incisal level and plane

Once the lower block is stable antero-posteriorly, it is necessary to ensure that the block meets the upper with bilateral simultaneous contact upon closure. Do not worry about the final occlusal vertical dimension at this point – just ensure that you have even contacts. Maintaining flat occlusal planes on each block by using a hot plate will ensure that this process is straightforward. Also, look very carefully for a slide – it is critically important to notice when this is happening, and to make necessary adjustments. Recording the relationship of the blocks *after* a slide is pointless and inaccurate. Your patient should be encouraged to close slowly and passively until they feel something touch. The aim is for even contact of the blocks – but if they stop short then you have identified an early contact – either between the heels of the denture bases, or between an uneven wax surface on one or both of the blocks.

Buccal relationship

The most stable masticatory position for the lower teeth is over the ridge. However, it is also important to consider the relationship to the upper teeth; normally we would expect the upper teeth to sit buccally to the lower teeth, in order to support the soft tissues effectively and prevent cheek biting. It is useful to transpose the upper buccal contour onto the lower block with a wax knife intraorally, in order to help you make the necessary adjustments.

Vertical dimensions, tongue space and speech

The final vertical dimension is a function of the upper block incisal level, the upper posterior occlusal plane, and the height of the complementary lower block. On the lower, typically we would expect the incisor tips to be just visible during speech, and the tongue to sit slightly superior to the lower occlusal plane at rest. The vertical dimensions are discussed in more detail in Chapter 23.

Once you have largely prescribed the lower block, it is useful to pare out the lingual aspect, to replicate the expected tooth contour. A 1 cm thick wax rim will severely restrict the tongue, causing displacement, and making assessment of speech very difficult. At this point, both the upper and the lower blocks should be anatomically similar to the intended tooth dimensions. This is the best opportunity to test the function of the blocks in terms of speech, paying particular attention to sibilant (s) sounds and fricatives (f). Whistling sounds indicate that the speaking space is restricted – whilst hollow 's' sounds indicate an excess of freeway space.

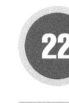

22 Tooth selection and arrangement

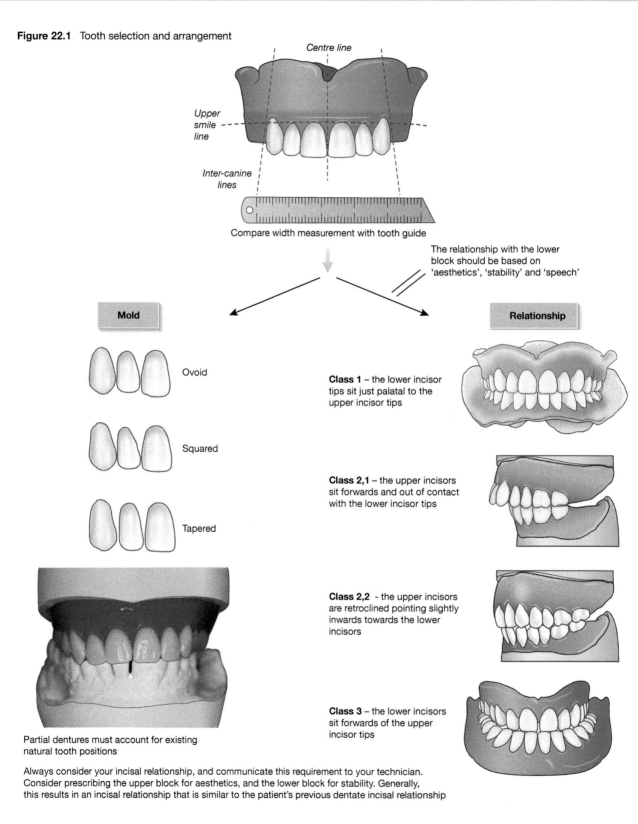

Figure 22.1 Tooth selection and arrangement

Centre line

Upper smile line

Inter-canine lines

Compare width measurement with tooth guide

The relationship with the lower block should be based on 'aesthetics', 'stability' and 'speech'

Mold

Ovoid

Squared

Tapered

Relationship

Class 1 – the lower incisor tips sit just palatal to the upper incisor tips

Class 2,1 – the upper incisors sit forwards and out of contact with the lower incisor tips

Class 2,2 - the upper incisors are retroclined pointing slightly inwards towards the lower incisors

Class 3 – the lower incisors sit forwards of the upper incisor tips

Partial dentures must account for existing natural tooth positions

Always consider your incisal relationship, and communicate this requirement to your technician. Consider prescribing the upper block for aesthetics, and the lower block for stability. Generally, this results in an incisal relationship that is similar to the patient's previous dentate incisal relationship

Removable Prosthodontics at a Glance, First Edition. James Field and Claire Storey. © 2020 James Field and Claire Storey. Published 2020 by John Wiley & Sons Ltd.
Companion Website: www.wiley.com/go/field/removable

The previous chapters have largely considered prescription of the upper and lower blocks based on soft tissue support and stability. Whilst both of these attributes can be *prescribed* by the wax blocks alone, it is also important to remember that the outer surface of the wax blocks is essentially your prescription for the placement of the denture teeth. This chapter therefore considers the choices surrounding tooth selection, and how you might define intended tooth arrangements.

An assessment should have been made prior to the commencement of treatment about the patient's aesthetic demands and requirements. It is therefore important at this stage to carefully revisit the treatment plan. It is not uncommon for patients to be unable, or find it difficult, to communicate their aesthetic concerns. Take the time to explore tooth arrangement and set-up at the planning stage. Does the patient want their prosthetic teeth to replicate their previous natural tooth arrangement? If so, do they have any photos that they can share? Prompt patients to ask whether they would like any 'gaps' between the teeth, or for teeth to 'overlap' (in relation to the overbite, overjet and imbrications). Clearly where natural teeth still exist, especially in multiple bounded saddles, the prescription will largely be determined by the existing tooth positions, shape and shade.

In the absence of any other useful information, it is possible to use biological guides as a starting point for planning tooth arrangements. A smooth and well-defined block (Figure 22.1) will facilitate this process, ensuring that your reference lines are clear to the technician.

Biological markers

The diagram in Chapter 20 shows the main biological guides to tooth arrangement. These include:
• The midline (which should correspond to the centre of the philtrum of the lip, or the nose)
• The high smile line (which is used to determine the cervical margin placement of the denture teeth)
• The canine centre lines (which should sit along a plane that passes through the inner canthus of the eye and the alar of the nose). This can be determined using a piece of dental floss.

A number of other anatomic features are purported to relate to ideal tooth positions, although there is little clinical evidence for this to be the case. If you are interested, I refer you to the recommended further reading to explore these concepts further. The overriding principle once again, is the interplay between aesthetics, stability and speech.

Tooth shapes

A huge variety of moulds are available for denture teeth and these largely centre around four main shapes – rectangular, tapered, ovoid and square. It is suggested that the category of tooth shape should largely conform to the patient's facial profile although in my experience there is often little correlation. It is important to consider the patient's wishes and expectations. The relationship of the blocks may also help you to suggest a particular tooth shape. I tend to find that an incisal Class 2,1 looks quite natural with tapered teeth and that ovoid teeth suit Class 2,2 relationships. If you cannot decide, try just setting the upper anterior

teeth initially. It is even possible to ask for a particular mould of tooth to be returned with your registration blocks in case you want to spend some time setting these up at the chairside. Whilst this takes a little longer, it can save an extra visit, especially if the patient decides they do not like the mould you have chosen. Having something to work from will usually prompt more useful thoughts or suggestions from your patient. Of course, if the patient is happy with their existing arrangements then you can use a stock tray to take an alginate impression of the current denture for the technician to copy. Whatever happens it is useful to give *some* indication to the technician that will help them to select a suitable tooth mould. Technicians often tell me that they are asked to set up teeth for a try-in where they are not even aware of the patient's sex. Clearly, the more information that you can provide, the better.

Tooth sizes

Whilst there are a number of shape styles available for denture teeth, most manufacturer tooth charts will allow even more specificity – this largely relates to the sizes of the denture teeth. It is helpful to the technician if you can at least estimate the intended tooth size. Most often this is conveyed on tooth charts as a distance around the arch between the distal surfaces of the canine teeth (Figure 22.1). Once the canine lines have been estimated, this can be measured with a flexible ruler. It is often said that the width of the central incisor should correspond to the width of the philtrum. Again, this is a rather sweeping generalisation – and in fact a lot of these measurements become futile if you are also asking the technician to set up teeth that are crowded or spaced. The main factor here is that you have prescribed the necessary anatomical lines onto the blocks.

Tooth shade and characterisation

Once again the patient should be directly involved in decisions about tooth shade. This process is somewhat easier for complete dentures, or where large anterior saddles exist, because this allows a degree of uniformity in relation to the apparent shade. The process is complicated by multiple saddles bounded by teeth with a disparate appearance. There really is no limit to the degree of characterisation that can be designed into a removable prosthesis – and given the time and technical skill, it is possible to create prostheses with a significant degree of camouflage.

Other considerations

Another aesthetic component that changes with age is the incisal level – the amount of incisor showing at rest and during speech. Typically this reduces as we age, and our facial tone reduces, with the incisors becoming increasingly 'hidden' behind the upper lip.

For complete dentures, or large anterior saddles, paring out the record blocks palatally and lingually will allow you to appreciate the incisor relationship that you are prescribing. It makes open bites and overjets more apparent. Ensure, however, that you explain to the lab which incisal relationship you wish them to set up, otherwise it is not uncommon for teeth to be returned for try-in with a Class 1 incisal relationship.

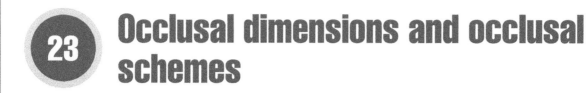

23 Occlusal dimensions and occlusal schemes

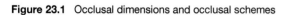

Figure 23.1 Occlusal dimensions and occlusal schemes

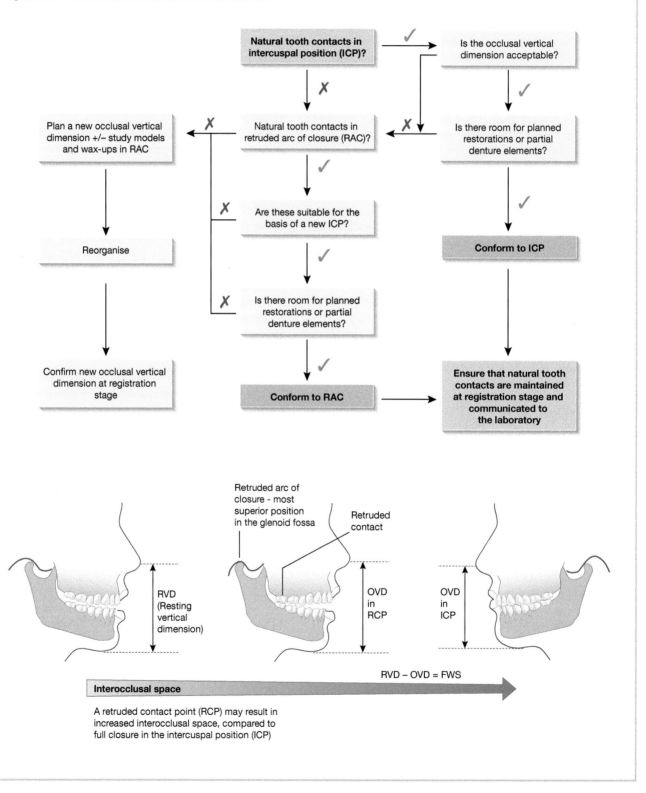

Removable Prosthodontics at a Glance, First Edition. James Field and Claire Storey. © 2020 James Field and Claire Storey. Published 2020 by John Wiley & Sons Ltd.
Companion Website: www.wiley.com/go/field/removable

This chapter aims to highlight several important aspects of occlusion relating to removable prostheses. The occlusal vertical dimension (OVD) for *complete dentures* is relatively straightforward to understand (Figure 23.1) – at rest, your patient should have a certain amount of 'freeway space' (FWS) between the teeth. This is usually expected to be around 2–3 mm but this is very much a guide. Your patient's existing FWS can be measured using a Willis gauge which sits beneath the nose and the chin. It is determined using the formula shown in Figure 23.1 – by subtracting the OVD from the resting vertical dimension (RVD). Callipers can also be used by taking measurements between a point marked onto the tip of the nose and the chin. Many factors can influence the results that you obtain (not least whether the patient has a big beard!) and so remember that this process is really just a guide. Determining that there is sufficient 'speaking space' is another useful process – and this relies on a qualitative assessment of the sounds that patients are able to reproduce, rather than a quantitative assessment of their face height. Wherever possible I prefer to use both methods.

Conform or reorganise?

Upon completion of your dental assessment for a *partially dentate patient*, your treatment plan will necessarily involve a decision about whether to alter the existing occlusal relationship (to reorganise), or to maintain it (to conform). The flow diagram (Figure 23.1) should help you to negotiate this decision-making process. Largely it will be determined by whether your patient has existing natural tooth contacts, and whether they occlude at a suitable OVD or not. If no natural tooth contacts exist, either in the intercuspal position (ICP) or the retruded arc of closure (RAC), then the process is actually quite straightforward, and involves prescribing the OVD at the registration stage. This can, of course, also be planned using a diagnostic wax-up on mounted study casts. On occasions, despite having stable natural tooth contacts, there may still be a need to increase the OVD – this may be required in order to:

- Augment the teeth with direct or indirect restorations
- Make room for partial denture elements such as rests or if an onlay design is to be used
- Restore the OVD to treat problems with overclosure such as temporomandibular joint disorders or angular cheilitis

In these cases, a new, *reorganised* OVD should be planned. This may become complicated if it is not immediately apparent how you might restore the existing natural teeth whose contact will be lost when the new prosthesis is fitted. Here, we rely heavily on the concept of the Dahl effect. It is not within the scope of this book to discuss this (or methods of recording the RAC further). The further reading section provides some links to useful articles and you will easily find information about the process in mainstream restorative texts.

Occlusal schemes

Our natural dentition is most often based on a 'mutually protected occlusion'. In the ICP the posterior teeth are loaded axially, whilst the contact on the anterior teeth is maintained only slightly. The stable posterior contacts prevent the anterior teeth from becoming overloaded, resulting in wear, mobility and drifting. As soon as an excursion (lateral or protrusive) is made, the anterior teeth take up the guidance. The posterior teeth disclude, which prevents them from being loaded non-axially. As such, the anterior and posterior teeth mutually protect each other.

When our patients have lost their posterior stability, you should consider how to replace this – the anteriors should be able to support the prosthesis and also allow guidance movements that cause posterior disclusion. Conversely, the opposite is true; with loss of anterior units, the posterior teeth should help to support a prosthesis, and the anterior units should be left out of full function in the ICP and yet able to provide guidance in excursions. Most of the time these occlusal features are overseen by your technician – however, it is important to be aware of these important principles when planning removable prostheses.

Anterior guidance is often divided into two schemes – canine guidance and group function (where more than one tooth is involved in guidance on any given side). In reality we rarely see unrestored patients with isolated canine guidance. That said, when we are designing a new occlusal scheme, guidance centred around existing healthy canine teeth usually provides a predictable and stable solution.

Where prostheses replace guidance teeth, it is important to consider which guidance pattern you wish to prescribe. Think about sharing guidance between natural and prosthetic teeth, and whether a prosthesis will benefit from any support around its guidance teeth to prevent them fracturing or wearing excessively. Cobalt chrome frameworks acting as backings to guidance teeth can be very useful.

Complete denture occlusal schemes

Traditionally it was thought that balanced occlusion was necessary to optimise the stability of complete dentures – canine guidance was avoided because it was felt that this caused instability and displacement. However, a number of comprehensive systematic reviews have concluded that the type of guidance prescribed for complete dentures has little effect on the patient's quality of life, or masticatory performance. If you anticipate that the patient will have a high degree of muscle activity, or there are severely resorbed ridges or fibrous tissues, then you might consider prescribing a lingualised occlusion. In this type of balanced articulation, prominent maxillary palatal cusps contact the mandibular central fossae, which acts to reduce interferences in excursion and more favourably distributes stress during parafunction.

Facebows

I am often asked whether a facebow transfer is needed. The facebow allows prescription of:

- The maxillary plane in relation to the temporomandibular joint hinge axis
- The distance of the maxillary teeth from the hinge axis
- The intercondylar width

These factors will all affect the excursive movements of the semiadjustable articulator, and are considered important if you intend to represent your patient's movements accurately and alter the OVD.

24 Respecting the neutral zone

Figure 24.1 Respecting the neutral zone

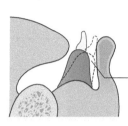

The neutral zone is a zone of passivity between the tongue and the lips or cheeks

There is often a discrepancy between the natural tooth position and the zone of neutrality

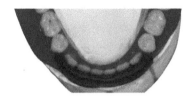

The neutral zone can be respected by:

- Paying close attention at the registration stage to labio lingual tooth positions in terms of stability and speech

- Recording the neutral zone formally using impression material

- Trialling alterations to labio lingual tooth positions at try-in by moving the teeth, or using carding wax to mimic new tooth positions (see image)

Recording the neutral zone

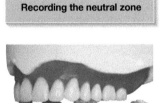

Use of a neutral zone tray, constructed at the intended OVD after the registration stage

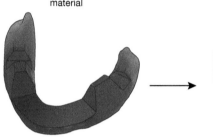

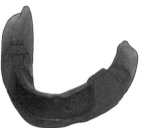

Notches cut ready to record the jaw relations

If a permanent base has been used, this lower block can be cut away, and the neutral zone recorded as part of the registration process

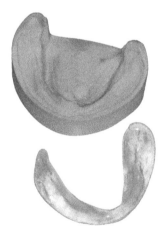

It is also possible to use a permanent base without any retentive features. Adhesive should be applied to the base, and a medium bodied silicone should be injected into the space between the lips, cheeks and tongue

Try-in

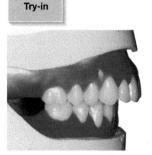

Note the overjet which is frequently prescribed as a consequence of respecting the neutral zone

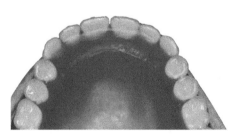

Placement of an anterior bite plane to account for the resulting overjet, can help maintain speech and masticatory function

Removable Prosthodontics at a Glance, First Edition. James Field and Claire Storey. © 2020 James Field and Claire Storey. Published 2020 by John Wiley & Sons Ltd.
Companion Website: www.wiley.com/go/field/removable

Another extremely common reason that lower dentures are unstable is because the denture is not sitting passively between the lower lip and the tongue. This area also involves the buccinator muscle of the cheeks and the orbicularis oris muscle anteriorly, particularly when patients are yawning or opening wide. We describe this passive area as the *neutral zone*. As described previously, denture instability can also be caused by base over- or underextension. It is very important to check that displacement is not exacerbated by these errors, before moving on to consider the neutral zone proper.

Diagnosis

With the lower denture in place, and the patient relaxed, the soft tissues of the lips and cheeks should be carefully retracted. If the lower denture still shows poor stability, lifts with tongue movements, or 'bounces' when fully seated, then it is likely that there are errors with the denture extensions. If the denture only displaces, particularly antero-posteriorly, when the soft tissues are allowed to rest back against the polished surface, then it is likely that the anterior teeth are not within the neutral zone.

Managing the neutral zone

Many classic texts and papers describe a specific impression technique to record the neutral zone, in order that the technician can place the denture teeth and polished surfaces in the most stable position. However, it is not always necessary to include a dedicated impression in order to account for the neutral zone. The following techniques can often be used in order to accommodate for the neutral zone without formally recording an impression.

Pay close attention at registration stage or try-in

When prescribing the lower block, pay attention to how stable it is in situ. Remove from the block labially if the block is displacing in a posterior direction (or remove lingually if it is displacing anteriorly). Note that if the block outline does not follow the contour of the arch, then this can also cause displacement from the neutral zone. This is particularly common around the premolar area buccally, where the modiolus is active. Aside from any corrections at the prescription stage, make sure that you pay close attention at the try-in. At this stage, it is not too late to alter the inclination of the lower anterior teeth, or to remove the lower anterior teeth and formally record the position of the neutral zone with an impression. The advantage here is that (assuming there are no overextensions and that the articulation is accurate) the patient is more able to carry out speech and swallowing functions than with the record blocks in situ. Furthermore, the material used for the neutral zone impression adheres more effectively to the roughened wax following removal of the teeth than it does to a smooth denture base.

Consider prescribing the anterior segment in carding wax

If you feel that you want to play around with some different tooth positions in order to find a zone of neutrality, then consider removing the anterior portion of wax from the lower block and replace with a thin piece of carding wax. This will allow you to make subtle changes antero-posteriorly to the wax work without having to spend lots of time adding and removing with hot wax. It is also possible to request that the blocks are returned without the anterior sextant waxed up in order for you to choose how you wish to record this zone. These are known as 'Manchester' rims, although you should be careful not to completely forget to prescribe the positions of the anterior teeth. Carding wax can also be used additively in order to help diagnose incorrect tooth positions or soft tissue support – both at try-in and when assessing existing dentures (Figure 24.1). When you are unsure, this saves removing teeth and spending time with hot wax; it can simply be removed again after testing.

The formal neutral zone impression

Ultimately, it may be necessary to use an impression material to record the neutral zone. This is often the case in particularly challenging cases, where the neutral zone is not created by a simple antero-posterior interplay between tissues. Examples of this include patients who have suffered a stroke, have a degree of paralysis, or have undergone surgery or laser treatment, and demonstrate restrictions because of scar tissue. The classic literature recommends the use of dedicated neutral zone trays (Figure 24.1) which are constructed after the casts have been articulated, and which sit against an upper try-in with occlusal stops. The trays can employ the use of wires or acrylic fins to help to support and retain the neutral zone impression material, but either way it is important to ensure that these features do not restrict free soft tissue movement, and affect the recording of the neutral zone. I tend to find that it is more accurate to leave a total void anteriorly (Figure 24.1). In fact, as a matter of routine, it is helpful to carry out the impression when you have finished prescribing the upper and lower record blocks. For this to be successful, you should ensure that you are working with permanent bases so that you can trim the wax entirely away from the anterior region without the block collapsing or distorting (Figure 24.1).

It is possible to use tissue conditioners as the impression material, but these are rather technique-sensitive and take a relatively long time to set. They also tend to slump and flow down around the tray extensions, which can be difficult to manage. I prefer using a medium-bodied silicone, which has a reasonable setting time, and can be easily trimmed back to the occlusal plane with a scalpel. Adhesive should be applied to the base, and this should then be placed in situ prior to syringing the material up the level of the occlusal plane. Do not worry, the material will be contained within the neutral zone. All functional movements including sipping water (early on to wet the mucosal surfaces) and swallowing, should be recorded. It is also helpful to ask the patient to say 'oo' and 'ee' in order to activate the modiolus.

The technician will make a putty matrix against the neutral zone impression before peeling it away and using the matrix to set the teeth. You can make this at the chairside instead if you wish.

Effects of respecting the neutral zone

You should once again be mindful of the interplay between aesthetics, stability and speech. If the lower anterior teeth are significantly distalised, it may be useful to prescribe a bite plane to facilitate sibilant and post-alveolar sounds. This can be waxed in by the laboratory for a try-in or by yourself using some carding wax (Figure 24.1).

25 Assessing trial prostheses

Figure 25.1 Assessing trial prostheses

Checks prior to trying in:

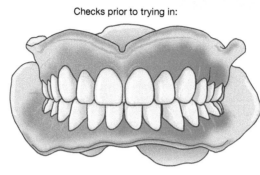

- Check the prescription in terms of mould, shape and size
- Check the incisor relationship, including overjet and anterior contacts

- Check for full base coverage
- Check for correct occlusal contacts and functional cusps (palatal upper, buccal lower)

For partial dentures, also check:

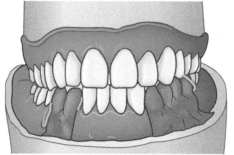

- Intended natural tooth contacts have been maintained
- Look for interferences from frameworks

- Look for unintended dead spaces
- Remind yourself of the path of insertion

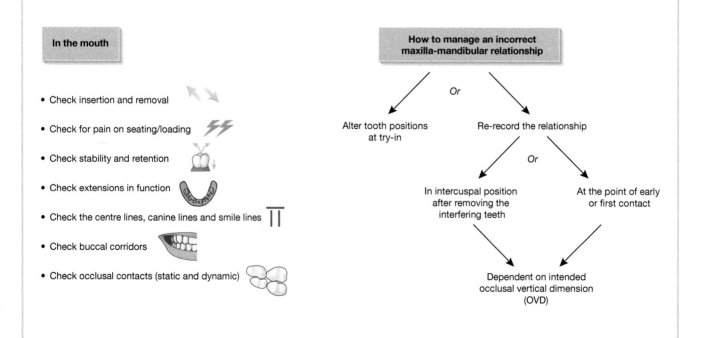

In the mouth

- Check insertion and removal
- Check for pain on seating/loading
- Check stability and retention
- Check extensions in function
- Check the centre lines, canine lines and smile lines
- Check buccal corridors
- Check occlusal contacts (static and dynamic)

How to manage an incorrect maxilla-mandibular relationship

Alter tooth positions at try-in *Or* Re-record the relationship

Or

In intercuspal position after removing the interfering teeth — At the point of early or first contact

Dependent on intended occlusal vertical dimension (OVD)

Removable Prosthodontics at a Glance, First Edition. James Field and Claire Storey. © 2020 James Field and Claire Storey. Published 2020 by John Wiley & Sons Ltd.
Companion Website: www.wiley.com/go/field/removable

Trying in prostheses should be a relatively uneventful stage, assuming that you have:
- Listened carefully to your patient's requests
- Correctly prescribed the intended tooth positions
- Considered the interrelationship between stability, aesthetics and speech
- Tested the function of your record blocks at the registration stage
- Accurately recorded the relationship between the upper and lower blocks
- Checked for the absence of heel clash (between casts or bases)
- Prescribed a registration record that can be reliably dismantled, disinfected and reassembled without ambiguity
- Communicated effectively with your technician

You may be daunted by this list – but be reassured that in all but very experienced hands, it is common for *something* to need at least minor adjustment – even if this relates to a minor heavy contact somewhere in the arch. Often, if you are struggling with the prescription stage, it is helpful to proceed to try-in. Errors are often more visible at this stage and are also often more easily corrected because the waxwork is less bulky, and existing teeth that can be moved or removed, as required. As mentioned previously, both the accuracy and success of the prescription *and* the try-in stage will be improved by using permanent bases.

What should be checked at try-in?

The short answer is: everything. All of the features and dimensions that you prescribed during your prescription and registration stage should be checked. Once again, the treatment plan should be revisited and discussed with the patient prior to trying the new prostheses. It is helpful to remind your patient about *why* they wanted new prostheses and the discussions you had about expectations, so that they can make a suitable comparison and judgement about whether they are happy to proceed to finish. Take your time and make it clear that beyond this stage there is little or no useful adjustment that can be made to the prostheses.

Features to check on the bench

- Try the prostheses on the articulated casts – check that the base extends across the full denture-bearing area and that the occlusal relationships are correct. This includes intercuspal and excursive contacts. On marking up, the functional cusps should be palatal on the upper and buccal on the lower (PUBL).
- For partial dentures, check that any expected natural contacts have been maintained and that the path of insertion conforms to your intended design, particularly in relation to guide planes and dead spaces. Pay close attention to teeth that have fractured off and have been glued back into place – these are risky areas where bounded saddles are concerned.
- For frameworks, check for unintended interferences such as excess wax around clasp arms or on the fitting surface.
- Check that the technician has followed your prescription for tooth position, incisor relationship, mould and shade.

Features to check in the mouth

- Check that the prosthesis can be fully seated easily without restrictions.
- Check that the occlusal relationships are correct. Once again this includes intercuspal and excursive contacts.
- With partial dentures that conform to existing natural tooth contacts, ensure that these contacts are maintained when the prostheses are in situ; try-in each arch independently first in order to more easily identify discrepancies.
- Check the extensions of the prostheses using functional border moulding and/or patient expressions, speech and swallowing.
- Load the prosthetic teeth axially in order to check for stability. Ideally you will have prescribed the teeth over the edentulous ridges where possible.
- Check soft tissue support, including the presence of buccal corridors, where necessary.
- Allow the patient to check the aesthetic outcome.

It is wise to allow the patient to wear the try-in prostheses for at least 10 minutes in order to be able to provide some meaningful feedback.

Managing occlusal discrepancies

You may notice a discrepancy when the prosthesis is in the mouth. This most commonly relates to an inaccurate registration, resulting in an early contact. This may result in a slide into an intercuspal position (ICP), a persistent open bite somewhere in the arch, or tipping of the prosthesis. Remember that in order to check for this, the patient should be relaxed, and you should assist them to close slowly until they feel something touch together. You should be in front of the patient to assess this and watch very closely as the arches close together. There should be no lateral or antero-posterior slide into the ICP. If a discrepancy is noted, you must decide whether you can correct it at the chairside or whether it is necessary to record the registration again and ask for a re-articulation and a re-try.

Heavy occlusal contacts that do not result in a slide or an open bite should be noted and adjusted at the fit stage – in my experience there tends to be a subtle degree of denture-base flexure and tooth movement during flasking and curing that often means the same discrepancies become elusive and are replaced by other minor discrepancies.

If the occlusal relationship has gross inaccuracies in the ICP, if the occlusal vertical dimension is incorrect, or there is a large slide into the ICP, then the try-in prostheses should be adjusted. This can be done three ways (Figure 25.1):

1 Tooth movement at the chairside.
2 Removing the interfering teeth, closing passively into the ICP and re-registering the try-in blocks together with registration paste.
3 Re-registering the try-in blocks at the point of an early contact (prior to a slide). This is technically more challenging and will undoubtedly result in a larger occlusal vertical dimension than was originally intended.

26 Fitting and reviewing finished prostheses

Figure 26.1 Fitting and reviewing finished prostheses

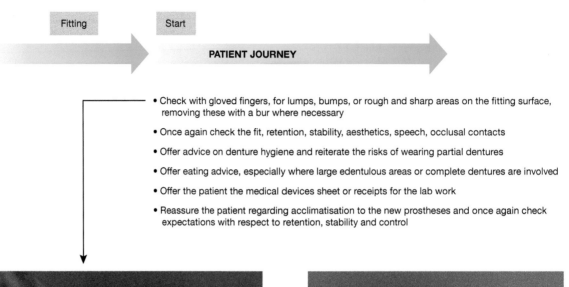

Fitting | Start

PATIENT JOURNEY

- Check with gloved fingers, for lumps, bumps, or rough and sharp areas on the fitting surface, removing these with a bur where necessary
- Once again check the fit, retention, stability, aesthetics, speech, occlusal contacts
- Offer advice on denture hygiene and reiterate the risks of wearing partial dentures
- Offer eating advice, especially where large edentulous areas or complete dentures are involved
- Offer the patient the medical devices sheet or receipts for the lab work
- Reassure the patient regarding acclimatisation to the new prostheses and once again check expectations with respect to retention, stability and control

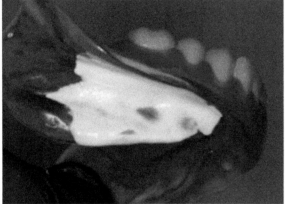

Pressure relief paste is applied to the fitting surface and the patient is encouraged to close into their intercuspal position

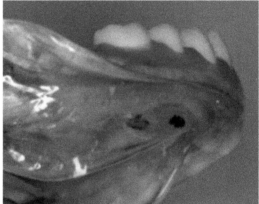

A soft pencil is used to mark thinned areas before the material is peeled off. Areas for adjustment are clearly visible

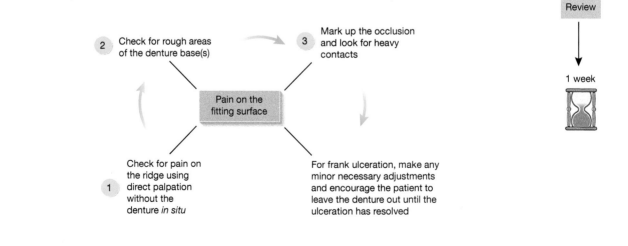

Review

1 week

2 Check for rough areas of the denture base(s)

3 Mark up the occlusion and look for heavy contacts

Pain on the fitting surface

1 Check for pain on the ridge using direct palpation without the denture *in situ*

For frank ulceration, make any minor necessary adjustments and encourage the patient to leave the denture out until the ulceration has resolved

Removable Prosthodontics at a Glance, First Edition. James Field and Claire Storey. © 2020 James Field and Claire Storey. Published 2020 by John Wiley & Sons Ltd.
Companion Website: www.wiley.com/go/field/removable

Assuming that the prescribed features of the prostheses were correct at the most recent try-in appointment, then there should be little of concern when fitting them. Nonetheless it is important to check the same features as you did during the try-in stage. This will include the fit, retention and stability, aesthetics and speech. It should not simply be *assumed* that the prosthesis will be satisfactory and it should always be fitted in the chair – never send it out in the post.

The fitting stage is an incredibly important event, not just because it is the culmination of the clinical and technical work, but because the patient is at the point where they will leave your surgery with the prosthesis in place. They should feel comfortable inserting and removing it and keeping it clean. They should also understand the risks to the oral structures if they *do not* maintain the prosthesis properly (this is discussed further in Chapter 44).

Note that we do not expect all patients to feel completely comfortable with the prosthesis in place – whilst for many this will be the case, it is the fitting stage where you should afford extra time and support to anxious patients, those who are wearing a prosthesis for the first time, or those who had experienced significant difficulties in the past. The more difficulties that you can anticipate and discuss with the patient in advance, the more favourably they will encounter them. They will also feel more comfortable with your advice and guidance, and also your reassurance. Sending patients away with unaddressed problems will damage your care relationship and may well result in patients seeking care elsewhere. If you do not see patients again, do not always assume you have been successful in your prosthodontic endeavours!

Some technical aspects will help you to anticipate and identify errors that need adjustment, and these are described below.

Returning on casts

It is a good habit to ask for finished prostheses to be returned on master casts (or if necessary, duplicated master casts). This can help you to identify errors that may have been introduced since the try-in stage, during processing. Before trying in the partial prosthesis you should remind yourself of your chosen path of insertion – this will help you to remove it from the casts, but also to insert and remove it confidently and effectively in the mouth.

On the casts, pay particular attention to areas of teeth that are worn, typically around bounded saddles. This can help you to identify areas that might be troublesome during fitting. It is then useful to place one sheet of thin (around 40 microns) articulating paper over areas of the dentition (either on the cast or in the mouth) before seating the prosthesis, to help you identify *specific* areas that may be binding. This is preferred to trimming away acrylic indiscriminately, leaving large embrasure spaces and defects, which attract food and plaque, and compromise retention and stability. If you have not prescribed a particular path of insertion for the partial prosthesis, then the technician will often process acrylic into a number of undercuts, expecting that you will make adjustments at the chairside. In this case it cannot be returned on a cast – ensure that adjustments are in relation to a single path of insertion only. It is *much* easier (and actually your own responsibility) to prescribe a path of insertion as part of your denture design.

Checking the fitting surface

If you are using permanent bases for complete dentures, then you may have carried this out at the prescription and registration stage. However, the fitting surface should be checked again, because it is always possible that lumps, bumps and sharp ridges of excess acrylic remain after processing. Prior to inserting in the mouth, spend a few moments running your gloved fingers and thumbs over the fitting surface. If any area seems sharp, then this should be adjusted with an acrylic bur. The surface should generally appear smooth without abrupt changes in contour. Small localised adjustments will *not* significantly affect the fit and stability of the prostheses. It is also possible to prophylactically investigate areas where the prosthesis is putting excess pressure onto the soft tissues – this can be done for complete or partial dentures and should be carried out using a closed-mouth technique. Pressure relief paste is rather technique-sensitive and messy to use, and so a silicone (light bodied or a specific pressure-indicator silicone) is recommended. A light wash should be applied to areas of concern, and the prosthesis seated fully prior to the patient closing into the intercuspal position. Areas of heavier contact can be noted and adjusted (Figure 26.1) with an acrylic bur prior to polishing.

Checking occlusal contacts

Once inserted into the mouth, you should re-check the occlusal contacts with thin articulating paper. Remember that the palatal cusps are functional on the upper, and buccal on the lower. Do not assume that this will be acceptable just because it was checked at try-in. Subtle changes during processing mean than small occlusal discrepancies often appear. Particularly heavy contacts will appear as a dark contact area surrounded by a lighter 'halo' – and these should be reduced slightly.

Reviewing the prostheses

I would recommend a review no longer than a week after fitting. Patients should be counselled that it is normal for some areas to feel a little sore. However, if the area becomes too painful or ulcerated and the prosthesis cannot be worn, then the patient should leave it out until the day before they come for review. Usually, sore areas on the fitting surface are because of a heavy contact. Marking up the contacts should be the *first* investigation that you make. Adjusting the fitting surface should be the *last* intervention that you make. All too often these are carried out in reverse! It is worth reminding patients that, paradoxically, successfully improving denture stability and retention has the potential to cause pain, as patients begin to use them more – the tissues will not be accustomed to being loaded so heavily or frequently, and so the greater the improvement, often the greater the expectation that there will be sore areas. Patients should be counselled about this and take it slowly – soft and small food items for a couple of weeks, and chewing at the back of the mouth. Patients need to understand that, in the same way that they would not run a marathon in new trainers, they need to build up their experience of wearing their new prostheses. A number of review appointments are normal, and patients should be reassured of this; it is not a sign of a failed construction process, *or* the inability of the patient to wear or tolerate them effectively.

27 Copying features from existing prostheses

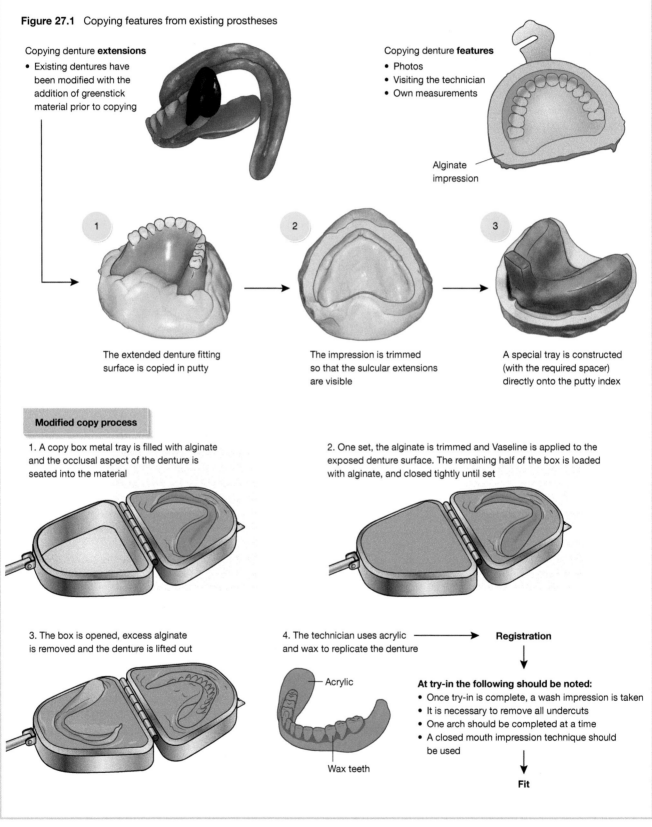

Figure 27.1 Copying features from existing prostheses

Copying denture extensions
- Existing dentures have been modified with the addition of greenstick material prior to copying

Copying denture features
- Photos
- Visiting the technician
- Own measurements

Alginate impression

1 The extended denture fitting surface is copied in putty

2 The impression is trimmed so that the sulcular extensions are visible

3 A special tray is constructed (with the required spacer) directly onto the putty index

Modified copy process

1. A copy box metal tray is filled with alginate and the occlusal aspect of the denture is seated into the material

2. One set, the alginate is trimmed and Vaseline is applied to the exposed denture surface. The remaining half of the box is loaded with alginate, and closed tightly until set

3. The box is opened, excess alginate is removed and the denture is lifted out

4. The technician uses acrylic and wax to replicate the denture → **Registration**

Acrylic

Wax teeth

At try-in the following should be noted:
- Once try-in is complete, a wash impression is taken
- It is necessary to remove all undercuts
- One arch should be completed at a time
- A closed mouth impression technique should be used

↓

Fit

Removable Prosthodontics at a Glance, First Edition. James Field and Claire Storey. © 2020 James Field and Claire Storey. Published 2020 by John Wiley & Sons Ltd.
Companion Website: www.wiley.com/go/field/removable

It is important to know how you might copy certain existing features of a prosthesis and this chapter considers various methods for doing so.

Tooth arrangements

One of the most common reasons for copying features is to communicate tooth arrangements to the technician – tooth mould, size, arch position and other characteristic features. The method involves taking an impression of the relevant denture teeth (usually the upper anteriors) within a stock tray. There is no need for a high degree of accuracy, and dimensional stability is unimportant, so alginate is the material of choice. Of course, it is also possible to take and send photos, or even communicate your own measurements – however, I find that an alginate impression is, in most cases, sufficient.

Fitting surface

If the current complete denture is largely correct, or you can easily make some reversible modifications, it is possible to copy the fitting surface in silicone putty. This can then be trimmed and used to make a special tray directly, which saves taking and casting a primary impression. The technique is especially useful if you are unable to access your usual impression materials – such as on domiciliary or other visits within a non-clinical setting. It is also dimensionally stable, which is important if the impression is going to be stored while you are out and about. Your technician should be instructed to construct a special tray in the usual way, 2–3 mm from the full sulcal border.

Full denture contour

Complete dentures can be copied in their entirety using copy boxes (Figure 27.1) which replicate the fitting, occlusal and polished surfaces. More often than not, however, we use copy boxes to create wax and acrylic replicas of the dentures, which are then modified clinically.

Modifying prostheses prior to copying

If dentures can be modified prior to copying their features, then it means there is less work to do at the subsequent stages. More often than not this involves additions to a denture that can be reliably carried out with greenstick or compound. This is removed once the impression has been taken. Waxes are a poor substitute because they tend to distort easily. Subtractive changes to existing dentures are less desirable and may be an indication to construct the new denture conventionally.

How to create modified copy dentures

Robust and rigid copy boxes should be used. Within each box, the occlusal and polished surface of the denture is seated firstly into alginate. Once set, the exposed denture and alginate are coated with Vaseline prior to the remainder being recorded. Once the denture is removed, and the box closed, this results in a void within which the copy template can be poured by the technician. Communication with the technician about which aspects you are intending to copy is critical to the success of the copy denture process. After copying, the dentures will be returned either completely in wax, or with acrylic bases and wax teeth.

You are essentially carrying out the recording of the jaw relationship next.

Registration

The wax teeth should be altered in order to obtain suitable tooth positions – if these were ideal in the copied dentures then there is little to do. The occlusal vertical dimension should be checked anyway, along with the occlusal planes and the incisal level and lip support. Because of the minimal amount of wax, this process is easier than with traditional blocks. The only drawback is that the copy bases are usually rather rough (they have been created from alginate impressions) and unretentive. Patients should be reassured that this is normal. Once you are happy, the copy blocks can be registered together in the usual way. Often they can be hand articulated, but it is better to verify that this is the case *in the mouth* first rather than making an assumption; just because the teeth interdigitate when hand articulated does not mean that this is an accurate representation of the jaw relationship in the mouth. Do not forget to prescribe a shade – and a mould too if you have altered the anterior waxwork so that the teeth are no longer visible. Often, when technicians copy dentures, they will also create a plaster cast of the tooth set-up so that they have a reference.

Try-in

The next stage is try-in – and this is essentially carried out in the same way as for conventional dentures (see Chapter 25). However, the main difference here is that once the try-in is correct, there is a need to carry out a wash impression (the major or working impression) in order to modify the relatively crudely copied bases. It is incredibly challenging to address the border extensions separately when they are constructed in wax; it is therefore very important to modify the denture, where possible, before copying. Crucial to the process is that undercuts should be removed from the internal aspect of the denture base. Inspect the base carefully and use an acrylic bur where necessary to trim back the base. If undercuts remain, then when the impression is cast, the denture becomes locked into place. The wash impressions are carried out using a closed-mouth technique. Each prosthesis should be loaded with impression material in the same way as a special tray – a thin icing of material (silicone or zinc oxide eugenol) in the internal fitting surface rather than being filled up. This ensures that the bases are seated fully. It also prevents a large inadvertent increase in occlusal vertical dimension, which is an unintended consequence of a closed-mouth impression technique when copying dentures. Each arch is taken in turn, and once loaded, the base is fully seated and the patient is encouraged into their intercuspal position. It is imperative that you continue to functionally border mould during the working impression – this is something that is often omitted, resulting in a copy denture which is overextended around the periphery. Once the impression material has set, the denture is left in situ, and the same procedure is carried out (as a closed-mouth impression) with the opposing arch.

Fit

The technician will process the try-in with the wash impression(s) for fitting at the next visit. The fit appointment is treated in exactly the same way as for conventionally constructed dentures (Chapter 26).

28 Classifying partial prostheses and material choices

Figure 28.1 Classifying partial prosthesis and material choice

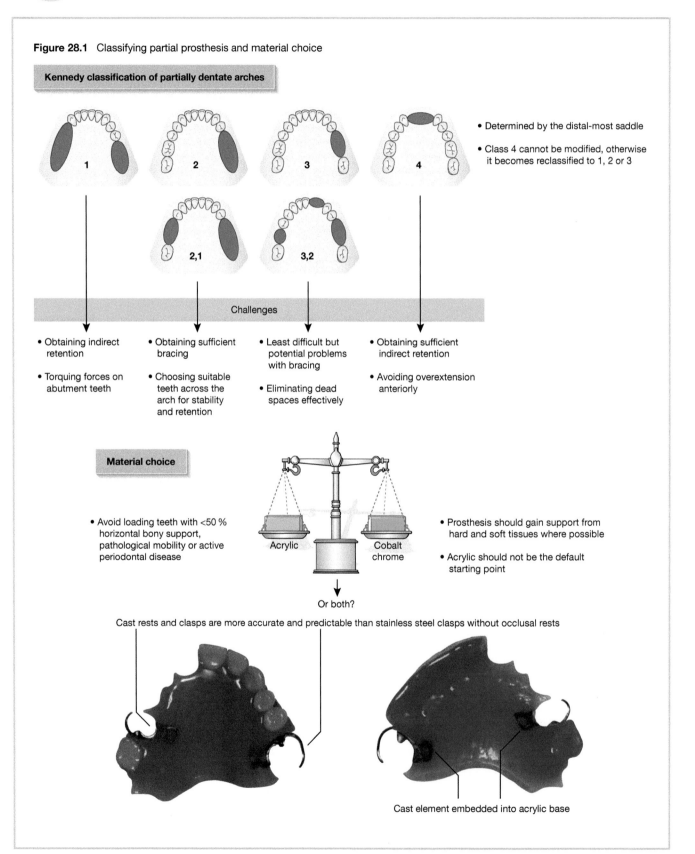

Kennedy classification of partially dentate arches

1 2 3 4

2,1 3,2

- Determined by the distal-most saddle
- Class 4 cannot be modified, otherwise it becomes reclassified to 1, 2 or 3

Challenges

- Obtaining indirect retention
- Torquing forces on abutment teeth

- Obtaining sufficient bracing
- Choosing suitable teeth across the arch for stability and retention

- Least difficult but potential problems with bracing
- Eliminating dead spaces effectively

- Obtaining sufficient indirect retention
- Avoiding overextension anteriorly

Material choice

- Avoid loading teeth with <50 % horizontal bony support, pathological mobility or active periodontal disease

Acrylic   Cobalt chrome

Or both?

- Prosthesis should gain support from hard and soft tissues where possible
- Acrylic should not be the default starting point

Cast rests and clasps are more accurate and predictable than stainless steel clasps without occlusal rests

Cast element embedded into acrylic base

Removable Prosthodontics at a Glance, First Edition. James Field and Claire Storey. © 2020 James Field and Claire Storey. Published 2020 by John Wiley & Sons Ltd.
Companion Website: www.wiley.com/go/field/removable

Classification systems for partial prostheses are taught within most undergraduate curricula – however, I find that for many, this knowledge is lost to the ether soon after graduation. This is probably because of a lack of engagement with the classification process in everyday clinical practice. It could be argued that knowing how to classify partial prostheses is largely an academic exercise – however, I would propose that it is useful to retain this knowledge for two main reasons:

1 In order to communicate with colleagues and make referrals appropriately
2 In order to identify some of the specific clinical and technical challenges that are associated with each classification

Kennedy Classification

This is perhaps the most ubiquitous classification. Prostheses are classified into four main classes, determined by the *distal-most saddle*. Figure 28.1 shows examples of each. A class can be modified by any number of extra, bounded saddles. Class 4 (a single bounded saddle that crosses the midline) *cannot* be modified – an extra more-distal saddle, in this case, would result in a different classification (with the anterior saddle becoming a modification of the new class).

Applegate Classification

This modification sees the introduction of two extra classes to the Kennedy system.

• *Class 5* – this is the same as a Kennedy Class 3. However, it recognises that the anterior teeth are incapable of providing axial support for the prosthesis.
• *Class 6* – this class suggests that the complete occlusal load can be entirely toothborne and supports the use of unilateral prostheses in some situations. I am not overly supportive of the concept of unilateral prostheses; these tend to be rather fiddly to seat into place and can suffer from a high degree of rotational forces when in situ because of the lack of bracing that they can obtain.

Potential difficulties with each class

• *Class 1* – bilateral free-end saddles – in these cases the biggest challenge is obtaining sufficient indirect retention to prevent the prosthesis lifting posteriorly. This means that the posterior denture extensions, the choice of connector and the clasping axis are critical. There is also potential to place a high degree of torqueing forces on the abutment teeth if the rest, clasp and connector assembly are not designed carefully. These concepts are all discussed further in subsequent chapters.
• *Class 2* – unilateral free-end saddles – in these cases the biggest challenge is obtaining sufficient bracing to resist displacement in function. Once again, the posterior denture extensions are critical – and, in the absence of any other saddles, choosing suitable and accessible natural teeth in the remainder of the arch to receive rests and clasps can be a challenge. There is potential with this class for the overeruption of opposing teeth to be more extreme than for Class 1; temporomandibular disorder is also more frequent than in Class 1.

• *Class 3* – bounded saddles – these cases tend to be the least challenging to restore. However, whilst there are often useful guide planes that can be engaged, it can sometimes be difficult to obtain adequate bracing, and to choose a suitable path of insertion that eliminates dead spaces effectively. This class is, however, potentially the healthiest in terms of hard and soft tissue support.
• *Class 4* – unilateral saddle crossing the midline – in these cases the biggest challenge, certainly in larger saddles that extend to the premolars or beyond, is obtaining sufficient indirect retention to prevent the anterior saddle dropping. It requires extreme care when prescribing the anterior borders to ensure that these are not overextended. It is also important to identify undercut on the anterior ridge, in order to decide to what extent a heels-down tilt for the path of insertion will provide an extra degree of direct retention.

Material choice

A partial prosthesis should, where possible, gain support from both the hard and soft tissues. This is considered to be the gold standard approach. A denture that employs a rigid substructure, such as cobalt chrome, allows this. The important caveat here is that hard and soft tissue support should be employed *where possible*. There are occasions where a completely acrylic denture is indicated, such as allergy to the metalwork, inappropriate/inadequate support from remaining teeth, or if the denture is to be provided as an immediate denture.

Periodontally involved teeth

As a rule of thumb, teeth that exhibit pathological mobility, over 50% horizontal bony loss, or active periodontal disease (deep, bleeding pockets) should be avoided when looking for tooth support. *All* teeth in the arch should be assessed in terms of their ability to provide support – and where possible, they should be considered. To provide a purely mucosa-borne denture (all acrylic) just because the patient has active periodontal disease is inappropriate.

If you do not wish to employ a full rigid framework, then it is possible to embed cast cobalt chrome elements into the acrylic base (Figure 28.1). Although this design is weaker than a full framework, you will achieve much better fitting and appropriately engaging rests and clasps than if wrought stainless steel is used. Stainless steel clasps often fail to engage tooth structure properly and are not accompanied by a rest. They distort easily and act with an abrasive action axially along the tooth (and potentially the soft tissues) as the denture is loaded.

Cost of rigid substructures

Cost is often stated as the main reason for not providing patients with cobalt chrome dentures within primary care. However, qualitative evidence shows that it is also a lack of confidence in terms of prescribing and planning for cobalt chrome dentures that prohibits their use. The following chapters will therefore aim to provide some clear guidance on tooth and mucosa-borne denture design.

29 Designing partial prostheses

Figure 29.1 Designing partial prostheses

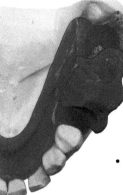

- Wax blocks used as carriers only
- Maintain natural tooth contacts passively
- Record the relationship of the block to the opposing surface using a silicone paste
- Fissures should be filleted out to prevent the casts bouncing on the highly accurate silicone record

- Record the coronal condition, periodontal status, bone levels and mobility scores of potential abutment teeth. It can be helpful to mark on the cast which teeth are suitable for providing axial support, or which to avoid as part of your design

- Send details of natural tooth contacts to the technician

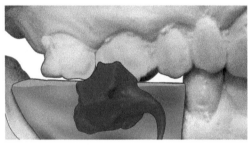

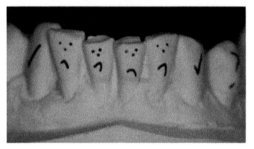

Design process

Step 1 – Eyeball the casts
- Classification
- Expected difficulties
- Dead space
- Undercuts
- Tooth arrangements

Step 2 – A system of optimal design

Step 3 – Surveying at the path of natural displacement (POND) and confirming a new path of insertion (POI) if required (chapter 32)

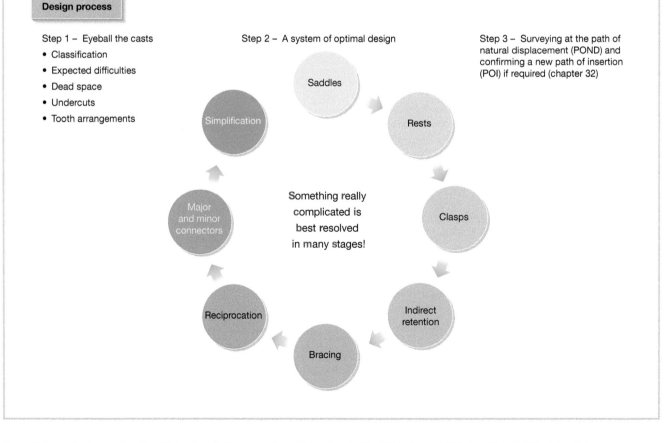

Removable Prosthodontics at a Glance, First Edition. James Field and Claire Storey. © 2020 James Field and Claire Storey. Published 2020 by John Wiley & Sons Ltd.
Companion Website: www.wiley.com/go/field/removable

The decision to provide partial prostheses should be derived as part of a wider and holistic treatment strategy, with the risks and benefits being explicitly discussed with the patient and recorded in the notes. This will necessarily entail a full restorative assessment – followed by a diagnosis, risk assessment and staged treatment plan. A template for this is provided in Appendix 2.

Preliminary registration

Once accurate primary impressions have been obtained, preliminary registration blocks (either on wax or temporary acrylic bases) should be constructed to allow you to record the intended relationship between the arches. More often than not, this involves recording (and maintaining) natural tooth contacts – but it may be necessary, even in the absence of tooth contacts, to assess the space between natural teeth and the opposing edentulous ridge.

This record is then articulated and will be used to inform your design process. This is arguably the least well executed aspect of partial denture planning and therefore you should check this articulation carefully – both at the chair side, before you send it to the technician, and when it is returned. It is useful to send details to the technician of the tooth contacts you have recorded in the intercuspal position so that they can verify the articulation. As described previously, the wax blocks should only act as carriers for a registration paste – and the process should be passive. Natural teeth should *not* be biting into wax blocks – you should hear the sound of natural teeth tapping together when the blocks are in place, nor should silicone be syringed around the entire arch. Cut definite and purposeful notches that will oppose natural cusp tips, and when the patient has closed into intercuspal position, syringe the material into the individual voids. Reassemble this at the chairside on the primary casts, checking for the intended contacts and also for interferences such as heel clash. It is useful to fillet out the fissures from the silicone registration with a scalpel to prevent this 'bouncing' on the less accurate primary casts. Alternatively, smear carding wax over the occlusal surfaces before taking the interocclusal record; the only detail you need to record is that of the cusp tips.

Other necessary information

In order to design an appropriate prosthesis that optimises hard and soft tissue support, it is necessary to consider some other factors:
• Recent periodontal indices (within the last 3 months ideally) to include pocket depths, clinical attachment loss, mobility scores and the patient's oral hygiene capabilities
• Recent radiographic assessment of potential abutment teeth (this can be obtained retrospectively when confirming the suitability of teeth to act as abutments if you prefer) in order to exclude any periapical pathology or root angulation that is not able to provide effective axial support
• Details of any coronal restorations for each tooth, including types of crown or inlay/onlay, details of direct restorative materials, pontic placement and support, and any planned replacements, refurbishments or *de novo* restorations.

Initially, it is useful to spend some time studying the casts – considering (without definite measurement) the classification of the prosthesis and any expected difficulties or challenges. I find it particularly useful to draw on the primary cast with a marker (Figure 29.1) in order to label or question the suitability of individual teeth to provide support or direct retention, or to highlight teeth that may benefit from further restorative intervention, such as new or replacement restorations, or restoration of tooth surface loss. Remember that individual periodontally involved teeth (those with active periodontal disease or pathologically mobile teeth) may be omitted from a design, whilst allowing other stable teeth to provide support. It does not have to be an all-or-nothing approach. The casts should ideally be mounted on a rigid articulator and be detachable – either by split-cast mounting or by using magnetic baseplates.

Other features that you should note at this stage include:
• Undercuts around teeth and edentulous ridges
• Severely tipped, tilted or rotated teeth
• Obvious dead spaces adjacent to saddles
• Embrasure spaces, particularly in patients with recession
• A lack of interarch space

A system of design

At this stage it is useful to sit down with a design template (Appendix 4) to work through a system of design.

At this point, many conventional texts will tell you to survey the casts. In the absence of any proposed design, this is a rather inefficient and laborious process. Practically, there is no need to survey *every* tooth surface in the arch – and trying to juggle all of the information yielded by this process can be extremely confusing. Instead, it is useful to come up with what you would consider to be an 'ideal' design, based on your initial examination of the cast(s) and the information listed above. This does make the assumption that you have adequate undercuts to clasp teeth and that guide planes or undercuts are favourable – but you can easily check this later. I find that this approach makes designing much more accessible and understandable for students. It also makes you quicker and more efficient.

I have devised a mnemonic to facilitate the design process. It ensures that you follow a logical, reproducible and comprehensive sequence. It is also a useful way of communicating a denture design, during an exam for example. Each aspect of design listed below should be considered, in turn, and drawn onto your design sheet. The following chapters will cover each in more detail, along with some specific case examples that highlight certain important principles.

Something **R**eally **C**omplicated **I**s **B**est **R**esolved (in) **M**any **S**tages

This stands for: **S**addles, **R**ests, **C**lasps, **I**ndirect Retention, **B**racing, **R**eciprocation, **M**ajor and Minor Connectors. The last stage is to consider whether your design is as simple as possible.

30 Saddles, rests and clasps

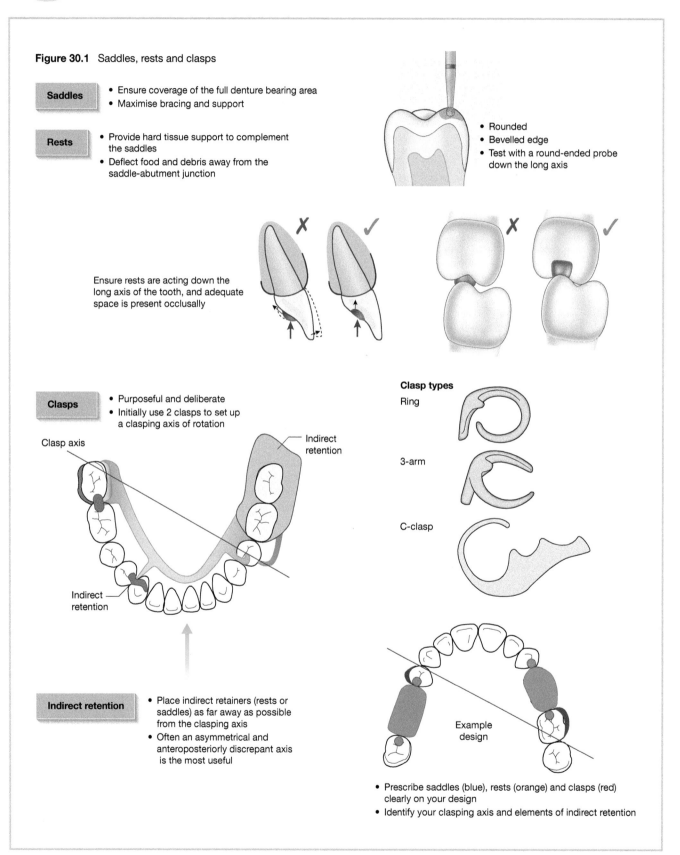

Figure 30.1 Saddles, rests and clasps

Saddles
- Ensure coverage of the full denture bearing area
- Maximise bracing and support

Rests
- Provide hard tissue support to complement the saddles
- Deflect food and debris away from the saddle-abutment junction

- Rounded
- Bevelled edge
- Test with a round-ended probe down the long axis

Ensure rests are acting down the long axis of the tooth, and adequate space is present occlusally

Clasps
- Purposeful and deliberate
- Initially use 2 clasps to set up a clasping axis of rotation

Clasp axis

Indirect retention

Indirect retention

Indirect retention
- Place indirect retainers (rests or saddles) as far away as possible from the clasping axis
- Often an asymmetrical and anteroposteriorly discrepant axis is the most useful

Clasp types

Ring

3-arm

C-clasp

Example design

- Prescribe saddles (blue), rests (orange) and clasps (red) clearly on your design
- Identify your clasping axis and elements of indirect retention

Removable Prosthodontics at a Glance, First Edition. James Field and Claire Storey. © 2020 James Field and Claire Storey. Published 2020 by John Wiley & Sons Ltd.
Companion Website: www.wiley.com/go/field/removable

Saddles

The first design features that should be prescribed are the saddles. This is where the prosthesis will derive its soft tissue support – and so it is important to consider covering the full denture-bearing area, particularly any distal extensions. However, prescribing a saddle for support does not always mean prescribing the replacement of missing teeth. A large saddle will usually provide a large amount of support and bracing, especially if you are able to engage the palatal vault and tuberosities on the upper or the disto-lingual and retromolar aspects on the lower. Do not forget that your ability to extend into these areas depends on how well extended your impressions were. Make sure that the saddles are drawn clearly, including the intended extensions (Figure 30.1)

Rests

Rests should then be considered. These serve three main functions:
• Complement the support offered by saddles, by resting on dental hard tissues
• Transmit occlusal loads from the denture down the long axis of the supporting teeth
• Deflect food away from the saddle-abutment junction

Most often, rests engage various aspects of the crowns of teeth – either small mesial and distal elements, larger shoulders or even onlay elements that restore large proportions of coronal structure. This support can also be obtained from sound retained roots, with an overdenture for example. As a rule of thumb, rests tend to be placed on either side of a saddle – but it may be the case, for short one- or two-tooth saddles, that only one rest is useful or, indeed, possible.

Rest preparations

You should check the articulation carefully to assess the relationship of the opposing surface to the intended rest position. Even if there is ample interocclusal space, a rest seat should still be positively prepared in order to ensure that it transmits forces down the long axis of the tooth, and that there is a seamless emergence of the framework from the tooth surface. Preparations should be rounded to allow movement in function. I recommend a large round diamond bur (1.5–2 mm diameter) seated to just over half its depth in the mesial or distal pit of the natural tooth (or equivalent place in an existing restoration). The bur should be carefully dragged down over the proximal surface in order to bevel this surface and remove any sharp line angles, and to make room for the framework to flow up and into the rest seat (Figure 30.1). Without this reduction the framework can end up bulky in this area, and at an increased risk of fracture because of sharp line angles. Check your preparation with a round-ended probe. The probe tip should be supported when loaded down the long axis. If it slips off, it is insufficient – the framework of the denture will suffer the same shearing action and fail to load the tooth axially. It is worth remembering that *sometimes* it is not appropriate to prepare a rest – the removal of sound tooth tissue or creating damage to an existing restoration outweighs the benefit of having a rest in that area. Your clinical judgement should be used in each case. That said, I would always consider whether existing restorations would benefit from replacement as part of the process. Porcelain-fused-to-metal crowns can be milled to

provide palatal or lingual shoulders, guide planes and undercuts for clasps. If you do choose to have crowns milled to a partial denture design, ensure that your technician leaves enough space for connectors rather than just milling guide planes and preparing rest seats in isolation.

Direct retention – clasps

At this point the directly retentive elements of your design should be considered. Primarily this will be derived from clasps, but also by engaging ridge undercuts – the latter is discussed in Chapter 32.

It is important to be deliberate in your prescription for clasps. Clasping excessive numbers of teeth will complicate the design, increase the difficulty with which the prosthesis is seated and removed, and result in greater amounts of food debris and plaque accumulating. As a rule of thumb, only two clasps are required. This is explained further, along with indirect retention, below.

Clasps will only be effective where the tooth surface is undercut in relation to both the path of insertion and the occlusal plane (path of natural displacement). This can be checked later on the surveyor. Clasps should always be supported by an occlusal rest – they are relatively fragile components and they should be passive when the denture is fully seated. The clasp tips should begin to engage at the point the denture displaces in an occlusal direction. Prescribing clasps without a rest means that the clasp arm can move up and down the tooth surface, causing distortion and trauma. Clasp arms need to be 'reciprocated' (balanced) to prevent displacement or jiggling forces on the abutment teeth. This can be achieved by the clasp encircling the tooth (ring clasp), another clasp arm on the opposite tooth surface (3-arm clasp), or the major connector itself (c-clasp) (Figure 30.1). At the surveying stage you should measure the depth of undercut to ensure that it is sufficient for the clasp to engage and to allow you to prescribe an appropriate material (cobalt-chrome 0.25 mm, gold 0.5 mm), or make modifications to the clasping teeth or your design. Generally, to avoid weakening the structure, gold clasps need to be embedded in acrylic rather than soldered to the cobalt-chrome framework.

Indirect retention

Generally, two clasps will enable a 'clasp axis' to be set up. It is about this axis that you should expect the prosthesis to rotate or tip. The clasp axis is akin to the centre point of a see-saw. In the same way that placing boxes under the end of the see-saw will stop it from tipping, rests, connectors and saddles prevent the prosthesis from tipping about its clasping axis (Figure 30.1). It is important to consider the elements that will provide the best indirect retention, on both sides of the axis. The further away from the clasping axis, the better the indirect retention. It is often best to opt for an asymmetrical and antero-posteriorly discrepant clasping axis, because this increases the likelihood that one of the indirect retainers is already in a useful position. Obtaining sufficient indirect retention is often a challenge with free-end saddles (especially bilaterally); ultimately the type of major connector, and whether rest elements can be placed onto any of the anterior teeth, become more significant considerations than in other Kennedy presentations.

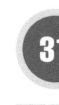

31 Connectors and bracing

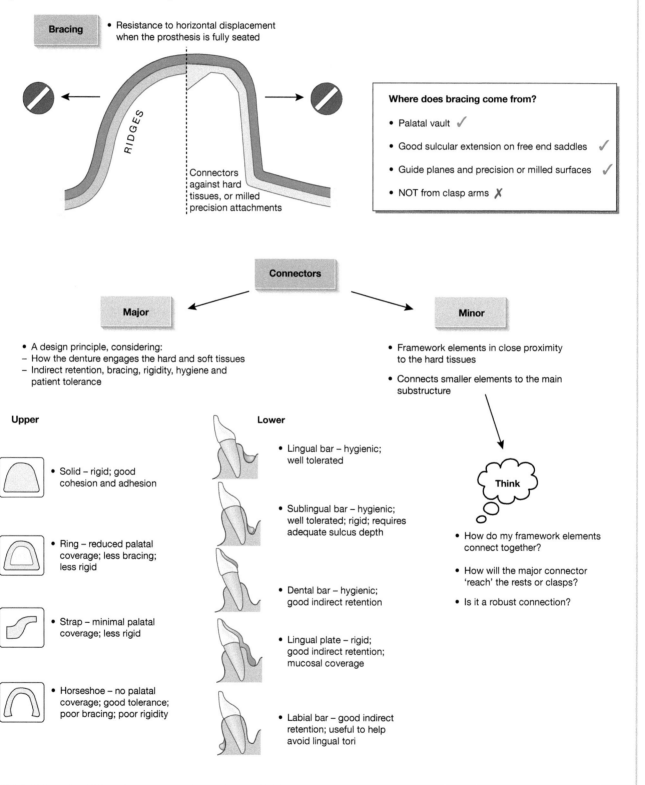

Figure 31.1 Connectors and bracing

Bracing

- Resistance to horizontal displacement when the prosthesis is fully seated

RIDGES

Connectors against hard tissues, or milled precision attachments

Where does bracing come from?

- Palatal vault ✓
- Good sulcular extension on free end saddles ✓
- Guide planes and precision or milled surfaces ✓
- NOT from clasp arms ✗

Connectors

Major

- A design principle, considering:
- How the denture engages the hard and soft tissues
- Indirect retention, bracing, rigidity, hygiene and patient tolerance

Minor

- Framework elements in close proximity to the hard tissues
- Connects smaller elements to the main substructure

Think

- How do my framework elements connect together?
- How will the major connector 'reach' the rests or clasps?
- Is it a robust connection?

Upper

- Solid – rigid; good cohesion and adhesion
- Ring – reduced palatal coverage; less bracing; less rigid
- Strap – minimal palatal coverage; less rigid
- Horseshoe – no palatal coverage; good tolerance; poor bracing; poor rigidity

Lower

- Lingual bar – hygienic; well tolerated
- Sublingual bar – hygienic; well tolerated; rigid; requires adequate sulcus depth
- Dental bar – hygienic; good indirect retention
- Lingual plate – rigid; good indirect retention; mucosal coverage
- Labial bar – good indirect retention; useful to help avoid lingual tori

Removable Prosthodontics at a Glance, First Edition. James Field and Claire Storey. © 2020 James Field and Claire Storey. Published 2020 by John Wiley & Sons Ltd.
Companion Website: www.wiley.com/go/field/removable

Once you have identified the hard and soft tissue support, and the retentive elements, you must then consider how to connect the components together. Even if you are unable to utilise teeth for hard tissue support, you may still wish to prescribe a cobalt-chrome substructure in order to reduce gingival coverage or to ensure greater rigidity and strength.

Bracing

At this stage it is worth considering your connector design and your bracing elements together; often the two go hand-in-hand. Bracing affords the prosthesis the ability to resist horizontal displacement *when it is fully seated*. This includes both lateral and rotational movement. Primarily, bracing will be obtained from base extension across the full denture-bearing area, and the ability to extend over ridges and into the palatal vault. Some degree of bracing can be obtained from minor connectors and rest elements, especially if they contain features that engage tall and broad vertical surfaces (such as a milled shoulder or a guide plane) (Figure 31.1); that said, it is best not to rely solely on these when considering how to optimise stability. Clasp arms do not afford any bracing, because the clasp tips should be passive when the denture is fully seated.

Major and minor connectors

Often, a source of confusion with rigid substructures is where a major connector 'ends' and a minor connector 'begins'. Actually, it is better to think of a *minor* connector as a design 'element' in proximity to the hard tissues which connects the finer or smaller elements, such as rests or free-end saddle meshwork, to the remaining substructure. As such, despite being called *minor* connectors, they still need to be robust enough to transmit load to both the underlying tissues and to the remaining substructure. *Major* connection, however, should be considered more as a design 'principle', which considers how the substructure should generally engage the hard and soft tissues, taking into account indirect retention, bracing, rigidity, hygiene and patient tolerance.

Minor connectors

When considering how clasps will be reciprocated, you should consider the mechanism for how the occlusal rest and clasp assembly flow from the major connector. When drawing your design onto the design sheet, make sure that you are explicit about how you wish each component to connect. Imagine the technician waxing up or designing your framework – is your design clear? Have you considered how a cobalt-chrome substructure will 'reach' each of your design elements whilst remaining robust? It is generally not a good idea to connect rests to other minor connectors such as saddle meshwork – ring clasps adjacent to saddles, for example, are probably best avoided.

Generally, frameworks should be at least 3 mm away from the gingival margins. Less than this, and the relatively small space encourages food-trapping and reduces cleansability. Conversely,

extending the framework up into the proximal spaces will increase the risk of gingival inflammation and root caries in the absence of meticulous plaque control; however, this approach can also offer a degree of indirect retention and bracing.

Major connectors

When considering how to connect the prosthesis across the arch, it is important to take into account the following factors:

• *Tooth spacing* – Any major connector sitting lingual or palatal to the crowns of the teeth will be readily visible if diastemata exist or the patient has experienced gingival recession.
• *Local soft tissue anatomy* – The presence of tori or shallow sulci may limit your choice of connector.
• *Clinical crown height and angulation* – Short or near-vertical palatal and lingual crown surfaces may offer little indirect retention or support.
• *Prognosis of the remaining teeth* – Anticipating future tooth loss in the short- to medium-term means that you may choose to bring a major connector closer to specific teeth.
• *Patient preference for mucosal coverage* – Patients who have previously worn a prosthesis may express a preference for gingival coverage. They may also demonstrate a strong gag reflex, which limits your choice of mucosal coverage. Where the posterior palate is causing a gag reflex, you may consider a horseshoe design – however, do not choose this route lightly. Gag reflexes are often exacerbated by poorly retentive and unstable dentures – plenty of reassurance and full coverage may be required. Nearly all patients will acclimatise successfully with this approach.
• *Patient oral hygiene capabilities* – The more complex the major connector, the less cleansable it will be and the more difficult it will be to keep debris and plaque-free.
• *The need for indirect retention, bracing and rigidity* – Extending a major connector onto specific anatomical areas such as the palatal vault or the lingual surfaces of the lower incisors may offer a degree of indirect retention and bracing, whilst also increasing the rigidity of the design.
• *The need to maximise cohesive and adhesive forces* – Increasing mucosal coverage across more of the full denture-bearing area will optimise cohesive and adhesive forces. This may be critical in difficult cases, such as Kennedy Class I and Class IV presentations.

The major connector choices are shown in Figure 31.1. Upper major connectors can take the form of solid connectors, ring-style connectors, strap connectors or horse-shoe connectors. Lower major connectors can take the form of lingual plates, lingual bars, sublingual bars, dental bars, labial bars, or labial and lingual bars concurrently. In my experience dental bars are significantly underutilised and provide a very suitable solution for patients who have embrasure spaces with a concurrent need for indirect retention in the lower anterior region.

Ultimately, the final choice relies on patient preference and your clinical experience – but do consider the full range of options on each occasion rather than defaulting to a habitual design or expecting your technician to choose.

32 Surveying and preparing guide planes

Figure 32.1 Surveying and preparing guide planes

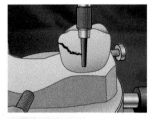

Marking a survey line on the cast

The provision of new PFM crowns with a clear path of insertion defined for the technician means that guide planes can be usefully employed – eliminating the need for clasps in this case

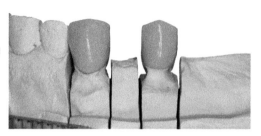

Assessing for guide planes

— Surveyor arm

The metal sheath of the surveyor arm protects the lead from snapping whilst surveying. The opposite side of the metal sheath can also be used for assessing dead spaces and guide planes

— Pencil lead

— Protective metal sheath

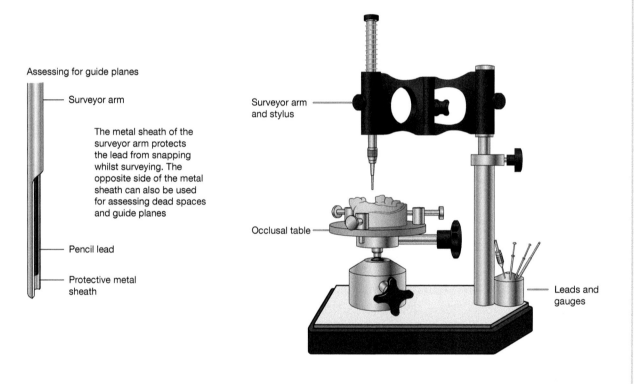

Surveyor arm and stylus

Occlusal table

Leads and gauges

Altering the path of insertion, where necessary, particularly in relation to engaging anterior saddle undercut

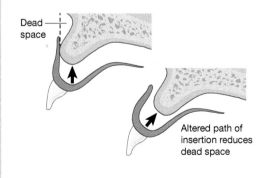

Dead space

Altered path of insertion reduces dead space

A method for communicating the chosen path of insertion to the technician. Three vertical marks are drawn onto the cast (bucally, mesially and lingually) in order to help re-orientation in the lab

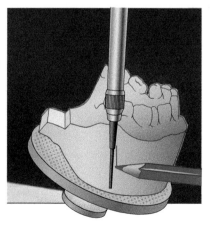

Removable Prosthodontics at a Glance, First Edition. James Field and Claire Storey. © 2020 James Field and Claire Storey. Published 2020 by John Wiley & Sons Ltd.
Companion Website: www.wiley.com/go/field/removable

Surveying is a critical part of the partial denture design process. As mentioned earlier, it is not always necessary to formally survey the casts *prior* to working through a design – in fact, for those becoming accustomed to the process, accounting for all of the information that an indiscriminate surveying process yields can often overcomplicate the design process and result in elements being missed or poorly considered. In my experience it also means that clinicians are less likely to consider other necessary tooth modifications such as restoring tooth form with composite or altering/replacing/providing indirect restorations with features that will complement the design such as shoulders, guide planes and relevant undercuts. Examining the casts before you begin, as discussed in Chapter 29, is still an important part of the process.

Should I survey for acrylic dentures?

Partial denture design is still very important even if you are prescribing an all-acrylic prosthesis. Base extension, gingival relief/contour and path of insertion (POI) should still be specifically prescribed. If you fail to prescribe a POI, then your technician may well process the acrylic denture into multiple undercuts, expecting you to make a decision and adjust the denture accordingly at the chairside. Unfortunately, to both you and the patient, it appears that the denture does not fit at all – and in an attempt to make it seat fully, you will often inadvertently remove acrylic from multiple paths of insertion – the denture will seat eventually, but it will be less retentive and stable, and with more dead spaces than if you had prescribed a single POI to the technician.

For rigid substructures, once you have an 'optimal design' it is time to survey the casts to check the feasibility. The following aspects should be considered.

Path of natural displacement

This is the direction in which the prosthesis will be inclined to displace in function – and is usually perpendicular to the occlusal plane. Surfaces of interest include teeth that you are intending to clasp (to check for suitable undercut), tooth surfaces adjacent to saddles (to check for dead space) and anterior edentulous ridges (to check for useful undercut to engage). The cast should be placed onto the surveyor table and adjusted until the occlusal plane is parallel to the bench top. A lead can be inserted into the surveyor arm – the lead is supported down one side by an extension of the arm, to prevent the lead from snapping whilst surveying. The lead should not extend beyond the metal support (Figure 32.1). The path of natural displacement can be traced laterally around the relevant teeth and ridges. The opposite, rigid side of the surveyor arm can be used to assess for dead spaces (Figure 32.1).

Path of insertion

You may wish to alter the POI from the path of natural displacement. This could be for a number of reasons, but primarily includes the desire to eliminate anterior dead spaces (often by tilting the heels of the cast away from the occlusal plane). On the upper arch this is known as a heels-down tilt. You may also wish to engage a greater degree of anterior ridge undercut,

or to engage specific guide planes that may exist. In the case of engaging anterior undercuts, your technician should only extend the denture to around 1 mm beyond the maximum undercut of a ridge. This may mean that, in relation to the path of natural displacement, the denture extensions are relatively short in this area, which will likely affect bracing, aesthetics, and food retention; therefore, engaging as much anterior ridge undercut as possible is recommended. It may also be necessary to alter the POI in order to negotiate tilted or rotated teeth.

Importantly, once you have chosen a new POI, the relevant surface should be surveyed again at the new path. For undercut to be useful, it must be *common* to both the new POI *and* the path of natural displacement. You then need to convey the new intended POI to the technician. Practically, a general description will often suffice (for example, a heels-down and slight left-hand tilt in order to reduce dead spaces and engage the anterior ridge – and to eliminate dead space on the left posterior bounded saddle). If the POI is more complex, then the new plane can be marked onto the casts using three tripod marks – bilaterally and anteriorly – to allow the technician to find the intended POI. It is still a good idea to explain both the altered POI and the rationale for your choice.

Guide planes

Employing two or more guiding surfaces can result in a prosthesis that is very retentive. In many cases, engaging multiple guide planes means that you can eliminate the need to prescribe clasps. Ensuring that guide planes are prepared appropriately is technically challenging. Guide planes should be at least 3 mm in height for them to be effective – it is therefore important to make sure the bur you are using is tall enough to cut the guide plane, and for you to make a judgement about the long axis of the bur at the same time. A long parallel-sided diamond fissure bur is a good choice – and at around 8 mm in length, you are able to assess the guide plane angulation relatively accurately. The more guide planes you decide to engage, the more technically challenging it is to directly prepare the surface to a single POI. One of the best ways to employ guide planes is to have them built into indirect restorations – the technician will be able to use a surveyor when waxing up the restorations (or use CAD software) to ensure that guide planes conform to a single POI.

Modifying the dentition

Once you have surveyed the cast(s) at the path of natural displacement and (if different) the POI, you are able to make a judgement about whether your optimal design will be possible. It may be that on occasions, a tooth you would like to clasp has little undercut. Here you have a choice – you can consider altering the clasping axis or consider altering the tooth itself. A tooth with little undercut can often be augmented with flowable composite (even crowns can be augmented if sandblasted and silane coupled first). You can also consider replacing crowns, and these should be replaced as porcelain-fused-to-metal designs with milled shoulders and guide planes where possible. The technician will need to know your intended design in order to make the new crowns first, and these should be fitted prior to taking the working impressions.

33 Designing frameworks – case examples

Figure 33.1 Designing frameworks – case examples

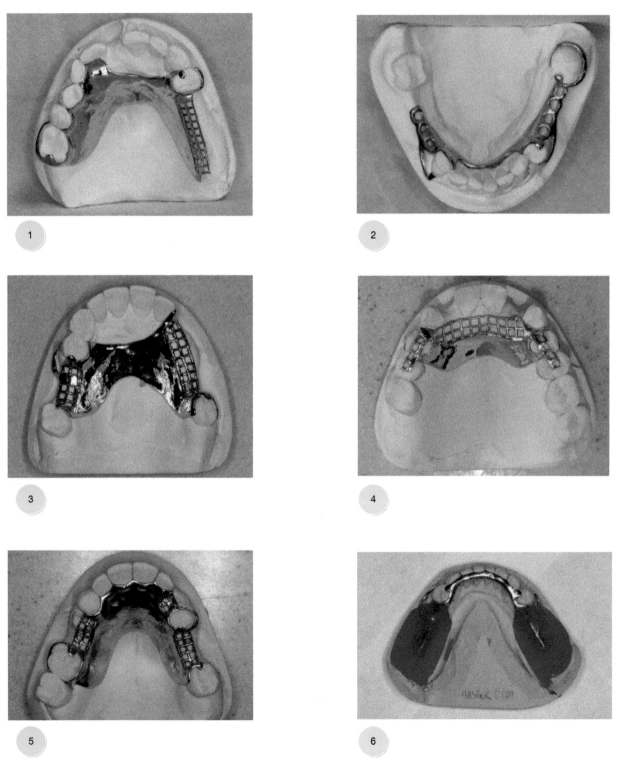

1

2

3

4

5

6

Removable Prosthodontics at a Glance, First Edition. James Field and Claire Storey. © 2020 James Field and Claire Storey. Published 2020 by John Wiley & Sons Ltd.
Companion Website: www.wiley.com/go/field/removable

The aim of this chapter is to identify and justify a number of design features by considering a selection of real frameworks at the try-in stage. These cases have been chosen because they raise useful discussion points, so feel free to discuss them further with colleagues and technicians. It is important to remember that there is unlikely to be one single ideal design – 10 dentists in a room will probably end up giving you 11 different framework designs. What is more important is that you are able to justify your design choices, ideally (in time) based on your clinical experience.

Example 1 – Upper Kennedy Class I, modification I

In this case, the clasping axis has been set asymmetrically and is antero-posteriorly discrepant in order to maximise the effects of indirect retentive elements, which should sit as far from the clasping axis as possible to maximise the mechanical benefit. This is an interesting case because of the large diastema between the centrals. If you are not careful and do not communicate the design properly, then your technician may be mistaken for assuming that you wish the small anterior saddle to be restored. The way the cast has been trimmed posteriorly is also slightly deceiving. The C-clasps on the premolar and the molar are accompanied by occlusal rests placed in accessible areas, and are reciprocated by the major connector in order to reduce the chances of clasp deformation. Indirect retention is obtained from the rests on the palatal aspects of the upper right lateral and canine, and the full extension across the ridge and around the tuberosity on the left. The rest elements anteriorly were also bolstered palatally to accommodate a relatively intrusive contact from the lower canine. The patient expressed a preference for a horseshoe connector design although it was possible to extend this slightly into the palatal vault to offer more bracing and rigidity. This meant, however, that it was not possible to relieve the framework from the gingival margins without compromising the rigidity. Extending up to the palatal aspects will improve the bracing element, although the patient must be aware of the increased risk of root caries and plaque accumulation if this is not kept clean.

Example 2 – Lower Kennedy Class III, modification I

In this case, the major clasping axis has once again been set asymmetrically and is antero-posteriorly discrepant in order to maximise the effects of indirect retentive elements. Indirect retention was considered on the lower left premolar and the lower right molar. The molar was periodontally compromised and unable to be utilised for hard tissue support and so as well as an occlusal rest for indirect retention, an extra direct retainer was placed on the lower left premolar. Ordinarily it is not a good idea to connect a clasp to another minor connector (the saddle meshwork on the left). However, in this case the undercut lingual to the molar was too significant to block out for a major connector and so a ring clasp was used to ensure reciprocation was present. This area of the framework will be particularly weak and it is important that the patient does not use the clasp arm to try and remove the denture. The direct retainer on the canine (i-bar) was reciprocated with a cingulum plate, which will also help with bracing. A lingual bar was prescribed because of imbrications of the lower incisors and the short clinical crowns.

Example 3 – Upper Kennedy Class III, modification I

In this case, the major clasping axis has once again been set asymmetrically although the antero-posterior discrepancy is limited by a requirement to avoid an unaesthetic clasp on the lateral incisor. This case is interesting because of the palatal torus, which prevented full palatal coverage from being prescribed. Indirect retention has been obtained as far as possible from the clasping axis, on the upper left molar and the upper right premolar. The C-clasps have been reciprocated with the major connector to ensure rigidity and aid bracing, given that the palatal vault is not engaged. The upper lateral was already crowned, and so a rest was taken up towards the distal aspect to afford the saddle some extra support, without having to prepare into the crown retainer. Another option would be to replace the crown with a porcelain-fused-to-metal (PFM) crown and to prescribe a tall palatal shoulder for axial support.

Example 4 – Upper Kennedy Class III, modification I

This case is interesting because a removable solution was being sought to address a loss of occlusal vertical dimension. The anterior teeth were restored with composite, but the premolar teeth failed to re-establish occlusal contact – the decision was made not to replace the existing indirect restorations. Instead, the framework was designed to allow onlay elements over the premolars. The patient's desire not to receive clasps on the canines, and the fact that the posterior restorations were not to be replaced, meant that the clasping axis, and the subsequent indirect retention, were compromised. The incisor teeth were of a dubious prognosis and so that anterior aspect of the major connector was perforated to allow future additions. You may wish to consider the benefits and risks of extending the framework posteriorly and up to the palatal aspects of the second premolars and first molars.

Example 5 – Upper Kennedy Class III, modification I

This case received new anterior crowns as part of the denture planning and design process. The PFM crowns had palatal shoulders to allow the framework to sit in close adaptation and be loaded down their long axis. The distal of the left lateral also had a guide plane prescribed, which corresponded to the medial of the premolar on the same side. The major clasping axis has once again been set asymmetrically and is antero-posteriorly discrepant in order to maximise the effects of indirect retentive elements. The patient expressed a preference for a horseshoe connector design although it was possible to extend this slightly into the palatal vault to offer more bracing and rigidity. The major connector was used in order to reciprocate the clasps, and there was little need to prepare a rest seat distally on the upper right canine because of the presence of a retained root, acting as an overdenture abutment. Indirect retention is obtained from the rest on the mesial aspect of the left molar and the palatal shoulders of the anterior PFM crowns.

Example 6 – Lower Kennedy Class II

In this case, the saddles have been restored using the RPI system (mesial rest, distal plate, i-bar) to reduce torqueing forces on the premolar teeth. Indirect retention has been optimised by placing a dental bar (which is further away from the clasping axis than a lingual bar would be). The advantages over a lingual plate are the reduced gingival coverage and improved cleansability.

34 Precision attachments – the fixed–removable interface

Figure 34.1 Precision attachments – the fixed-removable interface

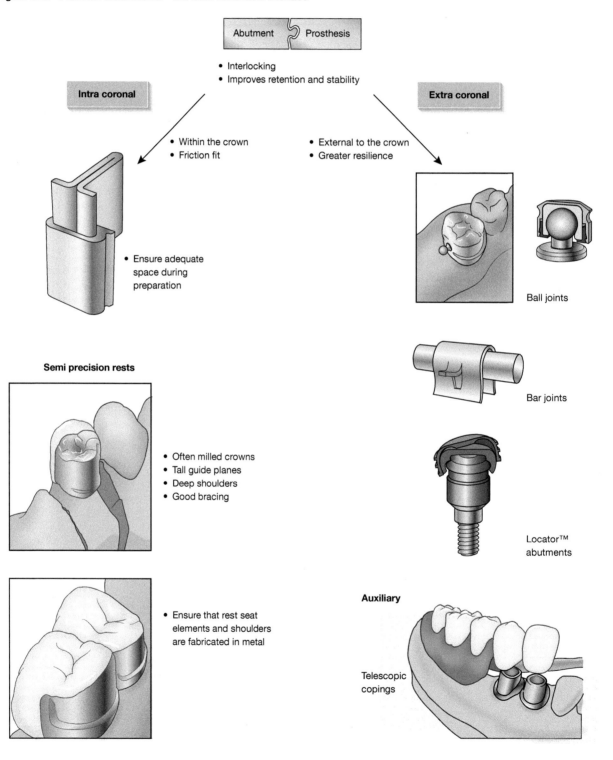

Abutment — Prosthesis

- Interlocking
- Improves retention and stability

Intra coronal

- Within the crown
- Friction fit

- Ensure adequate space during preparation

Extra coronal

- External to the crown
- Greater resilience

Ball joints

Bar joints

Locator™ abutments

Semi precision rests

- Often milled crowns
- Tall guide planes
- Deep shoulders
- Good bracing

- Ensure that rest seat elements and shoulders are fabricated in metal

Auxiliary

Telescopic copings

A precision attachment can be defined as an interlocking device – one component is attached to an abutment, and the other is part of a removable prosthesis. The primary aim of a precision attachment is to improve retention and stability of the prosthesis.

Employing precision attachments has, in the past, remained a relatively niche modality, requiring an able technician and a knowledgeable clinician who communicate well with one another. However, the art of intra- and extracoronal precision attachments is becoming increasingly accessible in relation to implant restorations, and with more manufacturers and technicians employing CAD-CAM, 3D printing, and laser sintering. Many mainstream companies such as Cendres + Métaux, Zest Dental Solutions and Nobel Biocare now offer a large range of precision attachment choices. Some of the most ubiquitous relate to mechanisms for improving the retention of removable partial dentures (RPD). Often these attachments consist of two matched precious metal components, although we are increasingly seeing resilient plastic components. One component is associated with the crown of the abutment tooth and the other is housed in the framework of the prosthesis.

Potential advantages of using precision attachments with a RPD
- Increased retention and stability
- Improved aesthetics (no visible clasping assemblies)
- Retention is unaffected by external coronal contour
- Reduced framework bulk
- Elimination of debris accumulation around clasps assemblies

Potential disadvantages of using precision attachments with a RPD
- Often requires more extensive preparation of abutment teeth
- Technique sensitive (clinical and technical) and is more time consuming
- Higher cost when utilising precision attachments
- Requires a minimum crown height (often >4 mm)

Classifying precision attachments
Precision attachments are most often classified by the attachment position.

Intracoronal attachments
Intracoronal attachments have the connection located within the crown of the abutment tooth. Generally, they provide a rigid connection between the abutment tooth and the prosthesis. Often this exists by way of a friction-fit mechanical lock. The degree of mechanical advantage this offers is related to the height of the clinical crown (and therefore the possible height of the intracoronal attachment). When employing intracoronal attachments, failure to prepare the abutment tooth with adequate space will result in a bulbous projection in the crown. Clearly this has implications for pulpal health and ideally should only be considered for teeth where large proximal restorations already exist.

Extracoronal attachments
As you would expect, extracoronal attachments have the connection (or part of the connection) located external to the crown of the abutment tooth. This means that the assembly tends to allow a greater degree of movement, or 'resilience'. The attachments most often take the form of ball joints, which project laterally from the crown. However, the attachments can also be studs (such as the Locator® systems), bars or magnets – and these tend to project occlusally. It is therefore important to ensure that there is sufficient space within the housing of the prosthesis (and within the anticipated occlusal vertical dimension) to accommodate these types.

The Locator® system is very popular as it offers a degree of resilience without the prosthesis completely detaching from the abutments. This is discussed further in Chapter 41, Implant-supported mandibular overdentures. Magnets are also still popular, especially on the faces of retained root abutments – however, resilience is poor and a small degree of occlusal instability can disassociate the magnet and its keeper. It can also be technically challenging to process the magnet keeper into the denture base accurately, so that it functions optimally. Therefore, magnet keepers are often 'picked-up' at the chairside once the prosthesis is completed, using cold-cure acrylic. Cobalt-samarium magnets are resistant to corrosion and can be processed up to 300 °C. Neodymium magnets are twice as strong and are very thin, but they must be coated to prevent corrosion and they will only tolerate temperatures of up to 150 °C.

Auxiliary attachments
The telescopic coping (or telescopic crown) is classed as an auxiliary attachment – because it is neither intra- nor extracoronal – it *is* the coronal aspect of the tooth (Figure 34.1). A thin metal coping of gold, cobalt-chromium or nickel-chromium is used to provide a durable outer coating to the preparation, which has an optimal total occlusal convergence angle. The prosthesis can be processed around the coping (either in acrylic or cobalt-chrome), or a sleeve can be manufactured which is picked up and embedded into the acrylic. The latter tends to be more durable.

A range of alternative attachments are also available, which cater for less common clinical presentations. In some circumstances, it is not possible to fit a removable prosthesis along one single and common path of insertion. In this case, it is possible to employ screw precision attachments to lock several pieces of the prosthesis together once fully seated. A similar and more accessible arrangement can be developed with bolts – a derivative of which is the swing-lock denture, described in Chapter 37. The advantage here is that with hinged flanges, it is possible to engage undercuts which would otherwise be blocked out, which improves the aesthetics, retention and stability, and reduces the incidence of food packing.

Semi-precision rests
Originating as the CSP (channel, shoulder, pin) system in the late 1950s, this approach – which required the fitting of a metal-based crown with guide planes, deep and tall shoulders and occlusal pin slots, upon which the framework would seat – became known as the 'milled crown'. More recent derivatives do not include the pin slots, but the guide planes and deep, tall shoulders provide remarkable bracing. These crowns should be porcelain-fused-to-metal-based, or all-metal, so that the seating framework can be afforded a degree of resilience without the risk of fracture of veneering material, or worse, fracture of the crown itself.

35 Dealing with frameworks and substructures

Figure 35.1 Dealing with frameworks and substructures

Cast rests and clasps

- More robust than stainless steel clasps without a rest
- More accurate fit
- Must prescribe a path of insertion for the technician

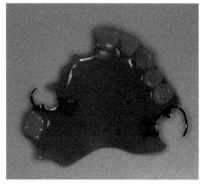

Alloy teeth

- Cobalt chrome or preformed stainless steel crowns
- Onlay elements to increase the occlusal vertical dimension or in bruxist cases to reduce accelerated denture wear

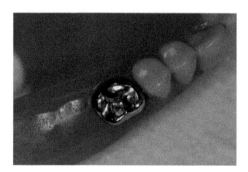

Accounting for additions

- If you are anticipating further tooth loss in the foreseeable future, plan for additions by asking for a perforated framework

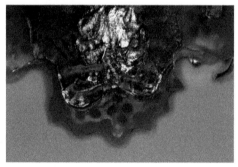

Try-in of the framework

- Check that your design has been followed

- Check your path of insertion

- Check for visible rubbing or wear on the casts

- Seat in the mouth, using the rest elements only

- Check the adaptation to the tissues

- Mark the fit surface with GHM articulating paper to identify binding areas

- Check the occlusion for interferences and aesthetics

Onlay dentures

- When designing onlay dentures, request bobbled frameworks in order to help retain acrylic or composite

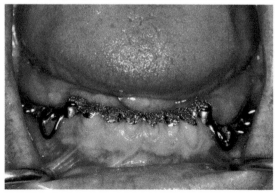

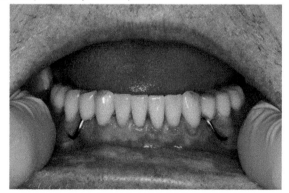

Removable Prosthodontics at a Glance, First Edition. James Field and Claire Storey. © 2020 James Field and Claire Storey. Published 2020 by John Wiley & Sons Ltd.
Companion Website: www.wiley.com/go/field/removable

Problems with rigid frameworks can cause a lot of frustration, primarily because they are relatively expensive, but also because problems with frameworks can delay treatment significantly because of turnaround times for re-makes.

Try-in of the framework

You may notice that the framework does not fit accurately. It is worth considering whether the working impression has distorted. This is most likely to happen if some impression material was not supported by the tray, the material has torn or peeled from the tray or there has been a dimensional change. These risks are reduced by using a silicone material. You may also have recorded distortions in tooth position if teeth were mobile or there was pressure on the teeth from the tray during the impression. Finally, air blows can be a source of error, so I advise pre-loading rest seats for a better result, either with silicone from a fine tip or with a smear of alginate. Do not assume that air blows can be 'flicked off' by your technician – just because they flick off, it does not mean that the area underneath corresponds accurately to the tooth surface.

• Check your design has been followed.
• Remind yourself of the path of insertion so that you can remove and place the framework back onto the cast and in the mouth without causing distortion or wedging.
• Check the cast for visible areas of rubbing, wear or fracture repair, because this will usually correspond to tight areas in the mouth.
• Attempt to seat in the mouth. If you feel resistance, seat thin GHM paper under the framework to mark-up tight areas. Look around rests and plates at the saddle junctions, especially around small bounded saddles. Make a decision about whether you can make any necessary adjustments or not. If not, you will need to retake the working impression, but do communicate the problems to the laboratory and send back the old framework as a reference. If seated fully, check that it is comfortable and that the patient does not feel any significant pressure on the dentition.
• Seat the framework using the rest elements only – avoid loading saddle areas, which will cause the framework to pivot.
• Check the occlusion – with accurate preliminary registration then this is seldom an issue, but if you have interferences, mark up with articulating paper in the intercuspal position and in excursions. If rests are becoming thin, then consider removing entirely or reconsidering a new design – thin rests will fracture and can remain very sharp.

Onlay dentures – Ask for bobbling so that acrylic or composite can be added, avoiding the need for labial flanges (Figure 35.1). If onlaying posterior teeth, you can prescribe cobalt-chrome if the patient has bruxist tendencies, or the acrylic is too thin to be retained effectively.

Cast rests and clasps – Using cast rests and clasps rather than stainless steel can be a cost effective alternative to a full cobalt-chrome framework, especially where just one or two clasps are required. The advantage here is that a rest can be included as a necessary adjunct and the rigid assembly works much more appropriately than a stainless steel wire, which is unsupported in function. In my experience these fit extremely well, but you still need to consider a path of insertion, dead spaces and undercuts.

Alloy teeth

These can be cobalt-chrome or stainless steel pre-formed crowns (Figure 35.1) – cobalt-chrome can be cast with engaging fins to allow the teeth to be embedded within the acrylic, or as mentioned earlier, as part of the substructure itself. Consider what material the denture teeth are opposing and whether the patient has bruxist tendencies or a particularly heavy bite.

Accounting for additions

As part of the denture design process, you should be considering teeth of short- to medium-term prognosis, that is, teeth that might be lost during the functional life of the prosthesis. In this case, it is worth designing frameworks that allow future additions (Figure 35.1), which may involve extending frameworks into areas that you might otherwise have left clear – and considering perforating the framework so that acrylic additions can be made easily.

Protecting small anterior saddles

On the upper arch it is common for single teeth or entire small saddles to fracture off the substructure. This is exacerbated in patients with deep overbites or parafunctional habits. It is worth considering in these cases whether you will extend the framework up onto the palatal aspects in order to protect these teeth in function. If there is no room to place a full prosthetic tooth onto the labial aspect, then it will most likely be trimmed down so that it veneers the framework in this area. If you can identify the need for this approach early, it will help you to design an appropriate framework and to check for occlusal interferences. This is where a preliminary registration is particularly helpful – and the technician may even want to send an anterior tooth try-in prior to framework construction, so that they can determine the ideal prosthetic envelope. This will help to inform your framework design – clearly in cases like this, it is of benefit to have an open dialogue with your technician.

Altering clasps

It is common for technicians to 'deactivate' clasps to facilitate seating and removal from the casts. This may lead you to think that the framework is unretentive or poorly fitting – and so it is important to inspect the framework on the casts in the first instance. The clasp tip should be sitting on the *surface* of the tooth, not away from it. You can ask your technician to 'reactivate' the clasp prior to finishing – but from time to time you may need to do this yourself – it is also necessary to adjust clasps over time as they distort, in order to re-engage with the tooth surface. Clasps should be adjusted with Adams pliers, and in my opinion it is much easier and more predictable to adjust a C-clasp that is reciprocated with the major connector, than a ring or a 3-arm clasp. Clasp arms tend to deform at their junction from the substructure, not within the clasp arms themselves. To avoid this, the tips of the Adams pliers should hold the clasp arm just prior to its junction with the occlusal rest – the clasp tip itself should not be adjusted. Do not grip too tightly otherwise the flat surface of the pliers will begin to flatten and distort the clasp arm. Instead, apply some gentle inward pressure. When you *think* you have seen the clasp tip move, that is enough!

36 The altered cast technique and the RPI system

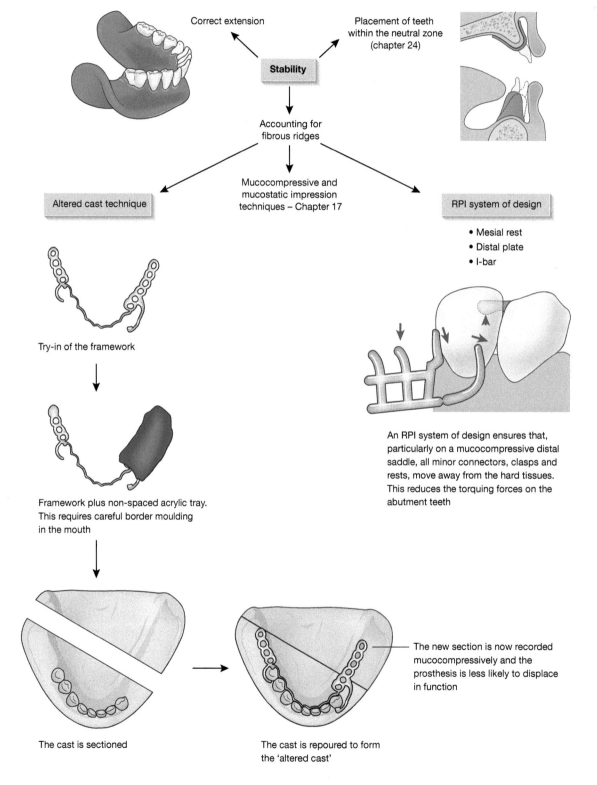

Figure 36.1 Altered cast technique and RPI system

Correct extension

Placement of teeth within the neutral zone (chapter 24)

Stability

Accounting for fibrous ridges

Mucocompressive and mucostatic impression techniques – Chapter 17

Altered cast technique

RPI system of design

- Mesial rest
- Distal plate
- I-bar

Try-in of the framework

Framework plus non-spaced acrylic tray. This requires careful border moulding in the mouth

An RPI system of design ensures that, particularly on a mucocompressive distal saddle, all minor connectors, clasps and rests, move away from the hard tissues. This reduces the torquing forces on the abutment teeth

The cast is sectioned

The cast is repoured to form the 'altered cast'

The new section is now recorded mucocompressively and the prosthesis is less likely to displace in function

Removable Prosthodontics at a Glance, First Edition. James Field and Claire Storey. © 2020 James Field and Claire Storey. Published 2020 by John Wiley & Sons Ltd.
Companion Website: www.wiley.com/go/field/removable

reviewing, we discussed strategies for optimising stability of a prosthesis. These included:
• Correct extension, both into the functional sulcus, and across the full denture-bearing area
• Placement of the teeth within the neutral zone
• Accounting for fibrous ridges

In relation to fibrous ridges, there are several approaches that can help to accommodate differential movement beneath the denture base. Respecting or compressing the tissues during a working impression was discussed in Chapter 17. This was largely discussed in relation to completely edentulous ridges. Whilst these techniques can be used in partially dentate patients, there are two other formally recognised techniques that can be employed. These are discussed below.

The altered cast technique

The altered cast technique can be used where the tissues overlying a free-end saddle are likely to cause downward displacement and rotation of the denture base in function. Accommodating for this displacement can reduce the torqueing effects of the framework on the abutment teeth. There is little evidence that this approach makes any perceived clinical difference – and using a relatively mucocompressive material during the primary impression can negate the need for any further special interventions. Regardless, if you decide to employ an altered cast technique to *formally* account for a compressive free-end saddle, this is usually carried out after the framework try-in stage. An extra appointment is therefore required. The aim of the technique is to 're-record' the free-end saddle mucosa with a greater degree of compressibility.

Once the framework accuracy is confirmed, the framework is adapted by the technician with an acrylic fin, which recreates the special tray extensions around the free-end saddle. No spacer is used by the technician when adding the fin; this means that when the framework is fully seated, and the acrylic fin is loaded with impression material, the impression becomes mucocompressive. Because the tray is not perforated, it is best to use zinc oxide eugenol, or a heavy-bodied silicone (with appropriate adhesive) to record the free-end saddle. Ensure, as normal, that the tray is adequately trimmed, and if necessary, border moulded with greenstick or putty.

Once the altered cast impression is received by the technician, the corner of the cast representing the free-end saddle(s) is cut away, and the framework is re-seated onto the model. The aspect of the model that is missing is then re-poured, to represent the compressed free-end saddle mucosa. In theory, the final prosthesis is less likely to 'bounce' in function and will reduce the torqueing forces on the abutment teeth.

A very common clinical mistake (and probably the reason that there is little reliable evidence for its use) is that the border extensions of the acrylic fin are neglected. Far too often the fin is simply loaded with material and the impression taken, without careful checking of the extensions or attention to border moulding. This results in a free-end saddle which is mucocompressive, yet overextended. One clinical problem is then replaced with another. *Do not forget to check the acrylic fin extensions, or to border mould adequately* during the altered cast impression.

It is also very important to ensure that you seat the framework by its toothborne elements *only*, otherwise the framework will tip when you load the free-end saddle(s). This is most likely with a Kennedy Class I presentation. If tipping occurs, it will result in a distorted cast when the impression is re-seated onto the working cast in the laboratory.

The RPI system

The RPI (rest, plate, I-bar clasp) system can also be used where the tissues overlying a free-end saddle are likely to cause downward displacement and rotation of the denture base in function. Instead of attempting to re-record the tissues compressively with an altered cast technique, the RPI system relates to a specific framework design that is thought to reduce the impact of denture base rotation on the abutment teeth.

RPI describes the following components, which specifically relate to the abutment teeth adjacent to the free-end saddle:
• Mesial *rest* (instead of a rest immediately adjacent to the saddle)
• Long distal *plate* (which engages from the marginal ridge down onto the attached gingival tissues)
• Gingivally approaching *I-bar* (which moves passively towards the embrasure space as the prosthesis rotates)

This clasping and resting combination is thought to reduce the torsional forces placed onto the abutment tooth. Ordinarily, with displacement over the ridge, a distal rest would place a non-favourable torqueing load onto the tooth, whilst a C-clasp tip would also engage towards the tooth surface rather than in an axial direction. Instead, a mesial rest and a gingivally approaching I-bar would move away passively from the tooth surface as the saddle is depressed (Figure 36.1). The distal plate *should* engage as a tall guide plane, which means that the distal aspect of the abutment should be prepared in line with the intended path of insertion. The long distal plate requires more meticulous oral hygiene because of its close contact with the tissues – however, it serves to stabilise the prosthesis further and to protect the tooth–tissue junction by preventing food impaction as the denture moves in function.

Often the RPI approach is only partially implemented – usually by way of a mesial rest and an I-bar. Once again there is limited evidence that the approach makes any clinical difference. I would certainly counsel against automatically prescribing this design for every free-end saddle that you come across. Pay attention to whether the free-end saddles seem to more be mucocompressive than normal. More importantly, you should consider where the occlusal rests can be *usefully* placed and employed, both in terms of any potential existing restorations, and in relation to the opposing occlusal contact(s). Blindly placing a rest mesially because of a free-end saddle is likely to cause more serious problems than a potential bouncing saddle!

37 Swing-lock prostheses

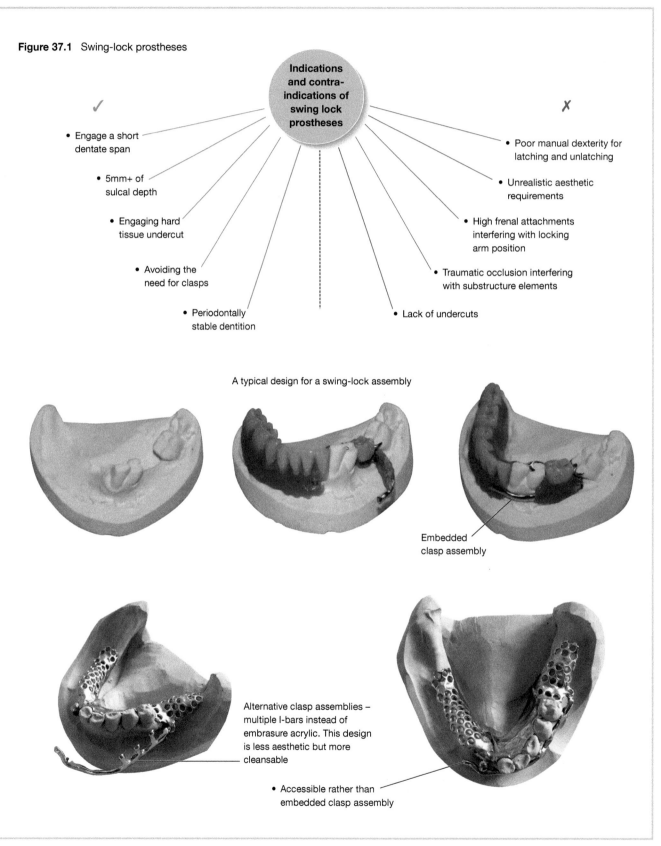

Figure 37.1 Swing-lock prostheses

Indications and contra-indications of swing lock prostheses

✓
- Engage a short dentate span
- 5mm+ of sulcal depth
- Engaging hard tissue undercut
- Avoiding the need for clasps
- Periodontally stable dentition

✗
- Poor manual dexterity for latching and unlatching
- Unrealistic aesthetic requirements
- High frenal attachments interfering with locking arm position
- Traumatic occlusion interfering with substructure elements
- Lack of undercuts

A typical design for a swing-lock assembly

Embedded clasp assembly

Alternative clasp assemblies – multiple I-bars instead of embrasure acrylic. This design is less aesthetic but more cleansable

- Accessible rather than embedded clasp assembly

Removable Prosthodontics at a Glance, First Edition. James Field and Claire Storey. © 2020 James Field and Claire Storey. Published 2020 by John Wiley & Sons Ltd.
Companion Website: www.wiley.com/go/field/removable

Swing-lock dentures tend to be labelled as specialist-level treatment. However, there is little reason why a swing-lock design should not be considered when planning treatment. With considered design features and good communication with a confident technician, they can be provided as part of the standard prosthodontic armamentarium.

What is a swing-lock prosthesis?

A swing-lock prosthesis consists of a preformed labial or buccal hinge, which attaches to a precision attachment, housed on the major connector. Traditionally, the swing-lock framework is cast as a single unit, although advances in polymer technology mean that 'replaceable inserts' are now available that can be embedded into keepers within the framework. Typically, a swing-lock prosthesis is inserted from the lingual or palatal aspect before the retentive bar closes across the labial surfaces. The retentive bar can engage undercuts provided by the teeth and/or the edentulous ridges, and is normally reciprocated by a lingual or palatal plate.

Indications

Some situations where you might consider a swing-lock design include:
• To engage short dentate spans, where at least 5 mm of functional sulcal depth exists labially
• A lack of support and retention for the prosthesis, such as hard tissue undercuts
• To avoid the need for prescribing or replacing crowns, or other extracoronal recontouring procedures
• To avoid the need for unaesthetic clasps or occlusal rests
• Where multiple embrasure spaces exist
• Where the prosthesis will gain support from a periodontally stable dentition

Contraindications

• *Poor manual dexterity* – Assessing the manual dexterity of your patient is incredibly important when considering a swing-lock design. This relates to their ability to insert the framework along a prescribed path of insertion, their ability to lock and unlock the latch assembly, and their ability to maintain meticulous oral hygiene around the abutment teeth. Swing-lock prostheses maximise their stability by covering the full lingual and palatal surfaces of the teeth – and so there is a significant risk of food stagnation, plaque accumulation and caries.
• *Aesthetic demands* – From an aesthetic perspective, it is also important to consider the height of the patient's smile line or position of the lower lip line. This will help you to determine whether any clasping or framework elements will be visible.
• *Frenal attachments* – Relatively high frenal attachments in the area of the framework should be viewed with caution. Adequate relief for these may compromise your design or completely inhibit extension of the framework into the length of the sulcus.
• *Traumatic occlusions* – Akerly Class 2, 3 and 4 traumatic overbites, or deep overbites, may prevent extension of the framework onto the full lingual or palatal surfaces of the natural teeth.
• *Lack of undercut* – A lack of undercut provided by the remaining dentition or alveolar ridges would mean that a swing-lock would fail to obtain any useful retention.

Assessing the periodontal condition

Some clinicians maintain that a swing-lock design can be useful for splinting periodontally involved teeth, especially because patients are transitioning towards edentulism. It is very important to counsel patients about the inherent risks of this approach – and whilst engaging the teeth may indeed help them to acclimatise to a removable prosthesis, it may *also* perpetuate or accelerate the deterioration of the engaged teeth. On balance, I would suggest that a swing-lock design is best employed around periodontally *stable* teeth (with no active periodontal disease); ideally with little mobility and at least 50% horizontal bony support. This is an arbitrary figure – and it is worth noting that in the absence of occlusal rests, and the presence of lingual plates, the axis of rotation is nearer the gingival margin. As such, there is minimal torqueing effect on the distal abutments.

The latch assembly

The latch assembly should sit in the recessive element of the labial ridge (Figure 37.1). You must ensure that the functional impression is accurate in this area – and this means careful extension of the special tray. I would recommend formally recording the border with a mouldable material such as putty or greenstick. Prior to the wash impression, any large embrasure spaces can be blocked out from the palatal/lingual surface, leaving some degree of embrasure engagement from the labial surface. This prevents tearing of the interproximal impression material and ensures good adaptation of the acrylic where required.

Retentive elements

The latch arm will be directly retentive as it swings closed and engages the ridge undercut. As described previously, it may also engage the embrasure spaces with acrylic (Figure 37.1). It is also possible to employ single I-bar type clasps (known as struts) or multiple struts (Figure 37.1). Acrylic veneering results in a much closer adaptation to the tooth surfaces, which results in better aesthetics (especially in cases with large embrasure spaces or recession) and less food packing.

In order to maximise bracing, lingual and palatal plates are taken up onto the lingual and palatal surfaces of the natural teeth, stopping short of the incisal surfaces. You may also consider occlusal rests on mesial *and* distal surfaces, and on multiple teeth. To optimise bracing further, porcelain-fused-to-metal crowns with guide planes and milled shoulders can be considered.

Connector design

Rigid connectors for swing-lock dentures can follow traditional connector designs, provided the lingual or palatal plate is present to act as bracing and reciprocation for multiple labial elements. In the maxillary arch, a strap, horseshoe, open palate or full coverage design can be successfully employed – although remember that a significant degree of bracing and rigidity will be obtained from engaging the palatal vault.

38 Gingival veneers

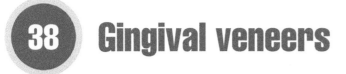

Figure 38.1 Gingival veneers

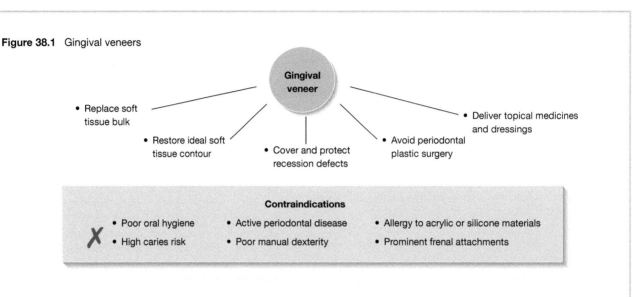

Gingival veneer

- Replace soft tissue bulk
- Restore ideal soft tissue contour
- Cover and protect recession defects
- Avoid periodontal plastic surgery
- Deliver topical medicines and dressings

Contraindications

✗
- Poor oral hygiene
- High caries risk
- Active periodontal disease
- Poor manual dexterity
- Allergy to acrylic or silicone materials
- Prominent frenal attachments

Addition of a tray handle, and the adaptation of the tray periphery anteriorly to engage the full sulcus contour

1. Accurate primary impressions, accounting for the full recording of labial surfaces and sulcus. It may be necessary to modify your primary impression tray, especially where more significant undercuts exist

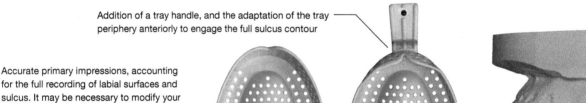

Stops

2. A special tray should be constructed that rotates around the canine tips, which will act as stops. Prior to taking the impression, palatal embrasure spaces should be blocked out to prevent through-and-through engagement of the silicone and subsequent tearing

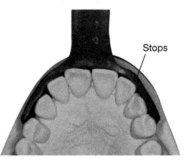

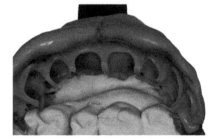

3. Shade recording using a gingival shade guide – this can also be determined digitally

The final veneer presented on the working cast

A gingival veneer (sometimes called a gingival prosthesis) is a removable device that is provided, most often in the anterior maxilla, in order to:

- Replace soft tissue bulk
- Restore ideal soft tissue contour
- Cover and protect recession defects
- Avoid periodontal plastic surgery
- Delivery topical medications and dressings to the periodontal and dental hard tissues

For most patients, the gingival veneer will address most, if not all, of these functions (Figure 38.1). Gingival recession can cause concerns over aesthetics, marked dentine sensitivity because of exposed root surfaces and problems with speech because of air escape through embrasure spaces. Some patients will also suffer from significant food accumulation and stagnation in larger embrasure spaces.

Regardless of the function(s) of the gingival veneer, there is no doubt that the patient's oral hygiene must be excellent. Such a close-fitting device will otherwise promote significant soft tissue inflammation and dental caries in the covered hard tissues. Many patients wearing a gingival veneer already present with exposed root dentine, which puts them at high risk of developing root caries, especially if the veneer is worn for long periods or if plaque and cariogenic substances have accumulated. Once the prosthesis is fitted, it is important to emphasise to the patient the need for regular review.

Contraindications

- Patients who are *unable to maintain excellent oral hygiene effectively* should be counselled against the use of a gingival veneer.
- I would also advise against the use of a gingival veneer, in all but the most temporary of applications, for patients with *active periodontal disease* or who have been assessed as having a *high caries risk.*
- Gingival veneers are relatively small prostheses that can be quite fiddly to fit and remove. Patients with *poor manual dexterity* may therefore struggle to manipulate the prosthesis – and, in my experience, I tend to find that *removal* is the most difficult aspect.
- If patients report or demonstrate an *allergy* to acrylic or any other denture-base materials.
- *Prominent frenal attachments* may weaken acrylic veneers, although this specific problem can be avoided by prescribing a silicone veneer. These present their own challenges and are discussed further below.

Veneering materials

Provisional or temporary gingival veneers can be fabricated directly in the mouth, or at the chairside, using silicones or light-cured sheet acrylic. This can be useful in order to provide the patient with an idea of the coverage that can be expected, or to provide an immediate solution. However, the aesthetic result using these approaches is likely to be unsatisfactory, and there are inherent risks of placing and curing acrylic material directly in the patient's mouth, both biologically and mechanically. Definitive gingival veneers are most often made indirectly and are constructed from heat-cured acrylic or silicone.

Indirect technique

A working impression is required that captures an accurate functional sulcus on the labial aspect. This may require the modification of stock trays and dedicated border moulding of special trays. It is important to block embrasure spaces (from the palatal aspect only) using carding wax, to prevent the impression material from locking into place and tearing on removal. A special tray should be constructed that sits on the incisal edges of the lateral and canine teeth, using them as stops. Light bodied silicone can be applied interproximally. The tray is then loaded with medium or heavy bodied material and rotated into place, which ensures a degree of sustained lateral pressure from the material into the interdental spaces. I would recommend avoiding putty, because this tends to drag when not completely confined by a closed tray. Removal should be linear, in a labial direction.

Retention

Retention for acrylic veneers is obtained by engaging the distal aspects of the canine or premolar teeth. A degree of flexion offered by the acrylic means that the prosthesis will 'snap' into place because it engages undercuts provided by the hard tissues. Once in place, the extensions into the embrasures (which replace the papillary form) will offer a degree of bracing and retention. A small degree of cohesive and adhesive forces from contact with the attached gingival tissues will aid in improving retention and stability. In more advanced cases it is possible to use *precision attachments* to connect gingival veneers to other fixed or removable prostheses in the mouth.

Silicone vs acrylic

Silicone veneers are becoming more popular, particularly as the degree of gingival characterisation improves. Whilst they are not as robust as acrylic, they can look more natural. Nearly all dead space is eliminated because the silicone can be withdrawn from undercuts. With silicone it is also possible to engage almost the full labio-palatal depth of the embrasure space. As a result, apart from helping with retention, silicone is useful for patients with crowded teeth, short dentate spans and for those with short bounded saddles. Silicone materials adapt more closely to the soft tissues in function – they obtain a significant degree of their retention from cohesive and adhesive forces. Patients who present with a dry mouth, and in the absence of any suitable saliva substitutes, may therefore struggle to manage a silicone veneer effectively. Furthermore, whilst silicone veneers show a good degree of adaptation and comfort because of their flexibility and close soft tissue contact, some patients report that they dislodge during eating more frequently than acrylic veneers.

Shade taking

Good communication with your technician is necessary from the planning stages onwards. Clinical photographs (including gingival shade tabs), diagrams and digital scans can help to communicate the architecture of the tissues, including the mucogingival line, stippling and vascularisation.

39 Immediate and training prostheses

Figure 39.1 Immediate and training prostheses

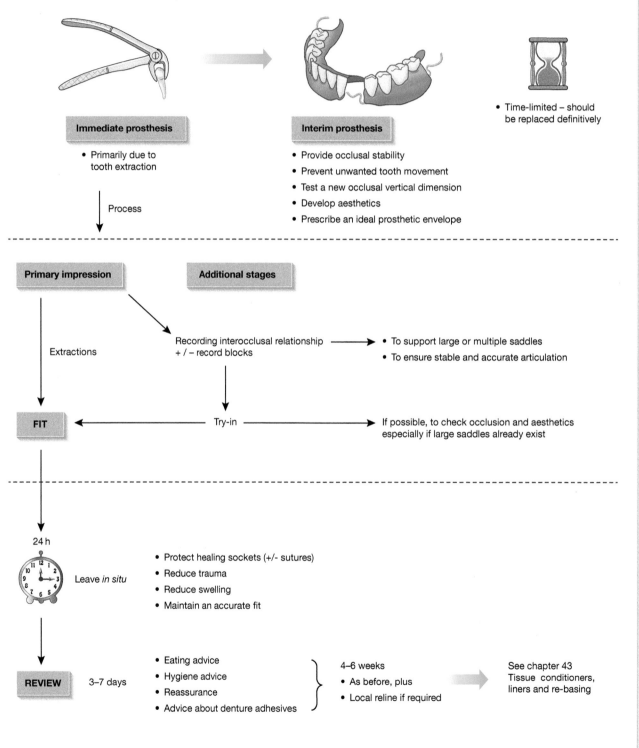

Immediate prosthesis

- Primarily due to tooth extraction

Interim prosthesis

- Provide occlusal stability
- Prevent unwanted tooth movement
- Test a new occlusal vertical dimension
- Develop aesthetics
- Prescribe an ideal prosthetic envelope

- Time-limited – should be replaced definitively

Process

Primary impression

Additional stages

Extractions

Recording interocclusal relationship
+ / – record blocks

- To support large or multiple saddles
- To ensure stable and accurate articulation

FIT ← Try-in →

If possible, to check occlusion and aesthetics especially if large saddles already exist

24 h

Leave *in situ*

- Protect healing sockets (+/- sutures)
- Reduce trauma
- Reduce swelling
- Maintain an accurate fit

REVIEW   3–7 days

- Eating advice
- Hygiene advice
- Reassurance
- Advice about denture adhesives

4–6 weeks
- As before, plus
- Local reline if required

See chapter 43
Tissue conditioners, liners and re-basing

Removable Prosthodontics at a Glance, First Edition. James Field and Claire Storey. © 2020 James Field and Claire Storey. Published 2020 by John Wiley & Sons Ltd.
Companion Website: www.wiley.com/go/field/removable

The Glossary of Prosthodontic Terms (published by the *Journal of Prosthetic Dentistry*) defines an immediate denture as one which is 'placed immediately following the removal of a natural tooth/teeth'. It may be a partial or a complete prosthesis. On occasions, a prosthesis also may be constructed with a temporary function, in order to provide occlusal stability, prevent unwanted tooth movements, test a new occlusal vertical dimension, or develop aesthetics; this is known as an 'interim' prosthesis. The interim prosthesis may also be immediate in nature. In any case, at some point both an immediate and an interim prosthesis should be replaced definitively. The process is outlined in Figure 39.1

Complete immediate dentures

Complete immediate dentures are commonly fabricated when a decision is made to extract remaining teeth in a terminal dentition affected by caries or periodontal disease, or where trauma has rendered the dentition unrestorable. They are usually constructed straight from a primary impression (Chapter 12), which might be challenging especially if the teeth to be extracted are pathologically mobile or painful.

The technician removes the remaining dentition on the stone models prior to fabricating the denture; as such, they make assumptions about how the alveolus will be modelled immediately after the extractions. It is not often possible or useful to have a try-in stage prior to final fabrication, because of the presence of the remaining natural dentition. It is for these reasons that the prosthesis may require some chairside modifications (usually by relining), or some denture adhesive in order to improve stability or retention. Aesthetics may also need to be modified anteriorly, both in terms of tooth position/mould and shade. To improve the fit, conveying the periodontal pocket depths of the teeth to be extracted can help the technician to estimate how much soft tissue collapse is expected.

At the fitting appointment, the patient must be prepared to acclimatise to the new immediate prosthesis – including leaving it in situ for approximately 24 hours post-extraction wherever possible to maintain stable blood clots in the sockets and to guard against swelling post-removal. If the prosthesis is left out, the patient may be unable to reinsert it or suffer considerable pain and distress doing so; it is worse if a large number of teeth are extracted or there are surgical extractions.

Denture hygiene instructions should be issued and advice regarding a softer, lighter, non-sticky diet avoiding overly chewy or crunchy foods. This is especially important whilst the person develops muscular control and is learning to function with their new prosthesis. Denture adhesive is useful in this learning phase. Three well-placed pea-sized blobs on the fit surface is usually sufficient, with instructions on how to remove the adhesive effectively from the prosthesis and the oral tissues. Patients are expected to adapt within 2–6 weeks but may need frequent adjustments and hard/soft relines during the healing phase.

A soft liner applied chairside can be useful to reline the denture during the healing phase. As the ridge continues to heal and remodel over approximately 6 months, multiple relines may have to be undertaken chairside to increase retention,

stability, confidence and adaption to the removeable prosthesis. Dependent on the number of teeth removed and the acceptability of the prosthesis to the patient, a hard chairside lining material may be considered if retaining it as a definitive prosthesis or a conventional remake of a complete prosthesis can be undertaken, correcting any features that have been unacceptable to the patient.

Partial immediate dentures

Where partial immediate dentures are to be provided following tooth extraction, wrought stainless steel clasps or Adam's cribs may be considered to aid retention because the prosthesis is *usually* entirely mucosa-borne – inaccuracies of immediate dentures at the fit stage normally precludes the prescription of rigid frameworks, unless the edentulous saddle in question is very small.

A pre-extraction impression is disinfected and sent to the laboratory, with a prescription clearly indicating which teeth are to be extracted, along with a shade – often the technician's judgement is used to match the shape of the natural teeth. An interocclusal record is required if there are no tripod tooth contacts remaining once the teeth have been extracted. You may require preliminary registration blocks to achieve this accurately.

Training prostheses

A training prosthesis can be provided to help patients to overcome barriers in adapting to a prosthesis. Most commonly this relates to hypersensitive gag reflexes, but it can also be very helpful when developing psychological acceptance of a removable prosthesis.

Training prosthesis are most commonly used on the upper arch, and usually consist of the baseplate component of a complete denture only. Sometimes several post dams are carved onto the prosthesis, allowing the clinician to sequentially nudge the posterior border more anteriorly with minimal loss of peripheral seal. In our opinion, it is more helpful to ensure the full denture-bearing area is covered, and for the patient to feel reassured and in control of the baseplate when it is in situ. In some respects, if necessary, it is better to work *towards* full palatal extension, rather than away from it. In any case, the baseplate should *always* be manufactured with a handle to ensure good patient control.

If the patient is able to tolerate mucosal coverage, anterior teeth (commonly canine to canine) may be added to the prosthesis, which may motivate the patient to persevere with the adaption process and restore some aesthetic aspects and social function. It is less common to offer a training plate on the lower arch – primarily because the main trigger zones for gagging are the posterior tongue and the palate.

The provision of a training plate will undoubtedly lengthen the treatment process – although it can prove to be an invaluable step in the rehabilitation of the patient. As with any acclimatisation process, the patient should be reviewed regularly, with plenty of positive praise as they develop their tolerance. It is not uncommon to see patients' personalities and presentations change dramatically as they overcome personal and psychosocial barriers to tolerating prostheses.

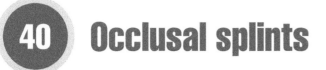

40 Occlusal splints

Figure 40.1 Occlusal splints

Preventing a traumatic overbite

Protecting restorations or rehabilitations

Managing temporomandibular joint disorder symptoms

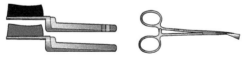

Occlusal splints
Permanent

Reducing bruxist sequelae

Testing increases in occlusal vertical dimension

Providing idealised occlusal contacts

1. Accurate full-arch impressions, which are well-supported by the tray

2. An accurate retruded axis record, at the intended occlusal vertical dimension

Wax should be thinned across the expected occlusal contacts

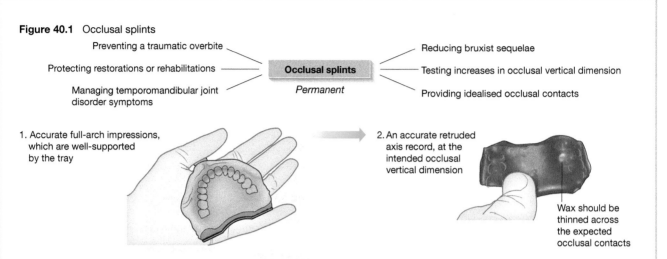

3. Mounted casts should be checked for accuracy and the intended occlusal vertical dimension should be verified or prescribed

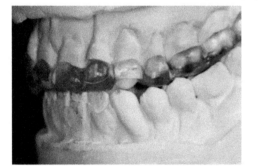

or

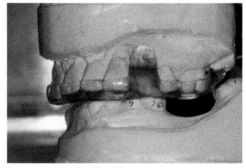

Maintain intercuspal position

Increase occlusal vertical dimension

4. Prepare materials and equipment for splint fit
- Millers forceps and GHM paper
- Shim stock and mosquito forceps
- Acrylic bur and high volume aspiration

5. The splint should seat fully without rocking or clicking into place
- Mark up tight contacts with GHM and make small adjustments until fit. Splints are typically tight interproximally and on the labial and buccal aspects
- Mark up retruded contacts, making adjustments until there are full arch simultaneous contacts
- Maintain a flat occlusal surface – do not create divots with the bur

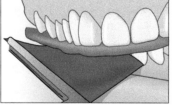

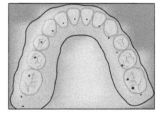

Adjustments are made with the lateral aspect of the bur to ensure maintenance of a flat occlusal table

- Mark up lateral and protrusive excursions and ensure there are no interferences
- Polish the splint prior to final fit
- Ensure the patient can insert and remove
- Arrange a review for no more than one week later

An occlusal splint is a removable appliance that is fitted to the occlusal surfaces of the maxillary or mandibular teeth in order to aid diagnosis or as a treatment intervention.

An occlusal splint may be fitted in order to:

- Reduce the impact of deflective or early contacts
- Provide idealised occlusal contacts
- Test increases in occlusal vertical dimension
- Reduce the physical impact of bruxist habits
- Manage the symptoms of temporomandibular disorder (especially if they exist *prior* to extensive or invasive plans for rehabilitation)
- Reduce the effects of a traumatic overbite
- Protect restorations both during and after treatment

A splint can therefore be considered as a *treatment platform*.

Splint types

The vast majority of splints made within primary care are *soft* splints. Typically, these are made from vinyl acetate, and are relatively easy to construct and fit. Most commonly they are made to fit the lower arch and are simply used to interrupt occlusal contact of the natural teeth. Soft splints are unable to be balanced because of their flexible nature – and adjusting them can be troublesome. It is therefore recommended that these are worn for defined periods only – such as during sport, during periods in the day when bruxist tendencies are likely, or overnight, in order to reduce the impact of sleep bruxism. It is important to note that soft splints may actually *exacerbate* bruxist tendencies and so, as with any removable device, arranging a review soon after fitting is advised.

The other main group of splints are *rigid* – these are primarily used as *stabilisation* devices in patients with unstable occlusal schemes, traumatic overbites or myofascial pain. These should provide firm and stable contacts in the intercuspal position, with canine guidance ramps for anterior guidance only. The occlusal surface should be as flat as possible to prevent intercuspation and encourage relaxation of the muscles of mastication. It is recommended that these splints are constructed in the retruded arc of closure. Typically, these are made from acrylic and are technically more demanding to construct, fit and adjust than soft splints. Stabilisation splints fitted to the upper arch are sometimes referred to as Michigan splints – and those fitted to the lower are also known as Tanner appliances. A review no later than a week after fitting is advised, because the majority of patients will distalise once their old intercuspal position is interrupted and further muscle relaxation occurs. It is therefore *nearly always necessary* to make minor readjustments at review. Other types of rigid splint include *anterior repositioning* splints that encourage the mandible into a protrusive position. This can be particularly helpful in patients with temporomandibular joint pain, joint noises or crepitus. A hybrid type of splint also exists with a rigid occlusal surface and a softer fitting surface. These are known as *bilaminar* splints and are purported to be easier to manufacture and fit. In my experience, however, this type of splint should be avoided where occlusal stabilisation is needed. This is primarily because although the splint may have a rigid occlusal surface, its softer fitting surface acts as a 'cushion' and allows the splint to tip and rock. This prevents the device from stabilising the occlusion effectively.

Occlusal coverage

It is extremely important to ensure that soft splints and stabilisation splints provide *full occlusal coverage* in order to prevent unwanted tooth movement and overeruption. This advice also extends to any other occlusal coverage device that remains in the mouth overnight or for long periods of time on a regular basis, such as bleaching trays. There are many instances where partial-coverage splints and trays have resulted in posterior overeruption and significant occlusal discrepancies, which can be quite complicated to manage. The best way to ensure full occlusal coverage is to extend the trays to capture the full arch. Remember to make sure that the impression material is fully supported, otherwise when poured up, the model will be inaccurate and the splint will rock antero-posteriorly.

Records for construction

Soft splints are often constructed using a single impression of the relevant arch. For rigid splints, accurate upper *and* lower impressions are a necessary starting point. They will then need to be articulated. It may be, especially if you have large or multiple edentulous saddles, that registration blocks are a necessity in order to help stabilise the interocclusal records. The interocclusal relationship should be recorded in the retruded arc of closure. The most predictable way to do this is to use *beauty hard wax*. This wax can be warmed and folded twice into a wafer. This should sit across the upper arch from canine to molar (Figure 40.1). Avoiding the incisor teeth reduces the risk of aberrant mandibular deviations on closing. The patient is encouraged to close into the retruded arc until the intended vertical dimension is reached. The wax is then cooled using the air syringe and removed carefully from the mouth. The wax is brittle when cooled, meaning that it is unlikely to distort without a noticeable fracture. If you have identified early contacts in the retruded arc of closure, these should be identifiable as the thinnest areas on the wax record (Figure 40.1). The cooled wax can be tried back into the mouth; the lower arch should close directly into the record, with a dull 'tapping' sound. Absence of this sound indicates the presence of a slide. In this case the record should be retaken.

You will need to choose a *vertical dimension* at which to construct the splint – this is often driven by the minimum amount of space that is required posteriorly (around 2 mm). Less than this and the splint is likely to fracture in function. There are two ways to prescribe the intended vertical dimension. The first way, with models mounted using a facebow on a semiadjustable articulator, is to increase the height of the incisal pin. My preferred method, however, is to record the intended vertical dimension directly intraorally as part of the wax record stage. This can then be mounted on an average value articulator without the need for a facebow record (unless further changes to vertical dimension are anticipated).

The clinical stages of record-taking and splint fitting are shown in Figure 40.1.

41 Implant-supported mandibular overdentures

Figure 41.1 Implant supported over-dentures

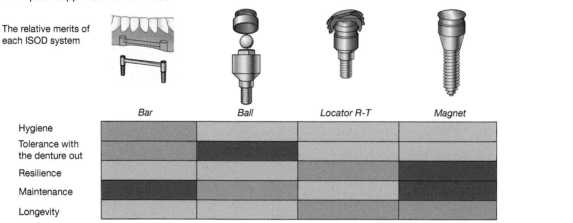

The relative merits of each ISOD system

	Bar	Ball	Locator R-T	Magnet
Hygiene				
Tolerance with the denture out				
Resilience				
Maintenance				
Longevity				

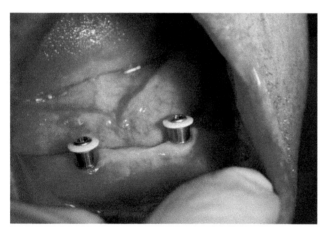

Locator abutments with the pickup rings *in situ*

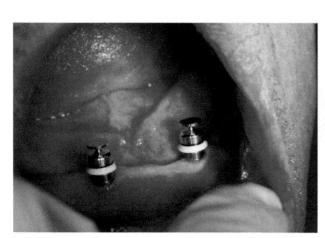

Closed tray impression copings *in situ*, ready to be picked up in the working impression

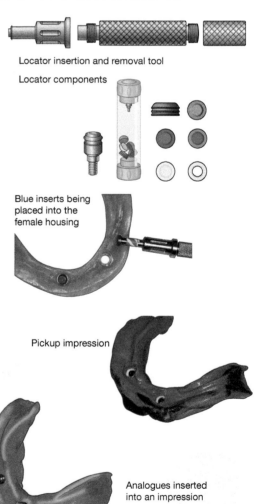

Locator insertion and removal tool

Locator components

Blue inserts being placed into the female housing

Pickup impression

Analogues inserted into an impression

Removable Prosthodontics at a Glance, First Edition. James Field and Claire Storey. © 2020 James Field and Claire Storey. Published 2020 by John Wiley & Sons Ltd.
Companion Website: www.wiley.com/go/field/removable

It is widely believed that implant-supported overdentures (ISOD) should be the first choice of rehabilitation in the edentulous mandible. A substantial body of evidence demonstrates that this is the case, both in terms of the patient's quality of life and from a cost–benefit perspective. Whilst you may not plan and place implants yourself, it is still important that you discuss ISODs with your patients as a potential treatment option. It is also important that you are at least *aware* of the stages required to plan, construct and maintain such prostheses.

Planning

Treatment planning should be prosthodontically driven. Therefore, the starting point is an optimal conventional lower denture which defines the intended prosthetic envelope (the zone within which the teeth are to be placed, in order to satisfy functional and aesthetic requirements). At this stage, the optimised prosthesis can be copied in a radiopaque acrylic and worn by the patient whilst a cone beam computed tomography (CBCT) scan is obtained. This will allow the planning clinician to take into account important anatomical structures such as mental nerve position, blood vessels and the quality and quantity of bone, in order to determine the optimal implant dimensions and angulations. It is not within the scope of this chapter to discuss further the stages involved in implant placement.

At the planning stages, it is important to choose and order the components for the attachment system that will retain the denture. Important factors for consideration include:
• Hygiene and cleansability
• Patient tolerance when the denture is removed
• Resilience (ability to withstand displacement prior to loss of attachment)
• Technical aspects of maintenance
• Longevity

If you require the attachments to be processed into the denture base by the laboratory (rather than picking them up at the chairside at fit), you will also require an abutment analogue, along with impression copings for the working impression stage. For ball and Locator® abutments, closed-tray impression copings are available – this keeps the working impression stage relatively straightforward.

Construction

Following well-extended primary impressions, a closed special tray should be requested with full coverage of the denture-bearing area, spaced for silicone and non-perforated. Space should also be provided above the healing caps for the abutment and impression copings to be attached.

The appropriate abutment height depends on the implant system and abutment system employed, and so you should follow the specific clinical guide provided. Locator® abutments should sit at least 1.5 mm clear of the gingival tissues. Knowing the height of the healing abutments is helpful in determining what size Locator® abutments to order. This can often be determined

from the clinical notes – if not, it may be necessary to remove them and measure them directly.

Polyether impression material is the most accurate and stable impression material for picking up ISOD abutments, although it is very rigid when set. With bars and divergent abutments, take care that the impression does not get locked into place. This can cause distress for both you and the patient when attempting removal. Undercuts should be blocked out with carding wax prior to taking the impression.

The special tray should be adjusted and border moulded with the ISOD abutments in situ. The same principles apply as for conventional dentures (Chapter 16). Once complete, laboratory analogues should be seated into the impression copings at the chairside to ensure that they are adequately and accurately seated (Figure 41.1). Requesting a permanent base for recording the jaw relations and subsequent try-in stage means that you are able to maximise the retention of the denture base during these critical stages and improve accuracy.

When fitting the prosthesis, the female retentive component may require activation. The manufacturer's instructions should be followed and appropriate tools used. Where Locator® abutments are employed, care should be taken when seating to ensure that the peripheral plastic does not fold over and prevent full engagement. You may consider using Locator R-Tx inserts, which not only account for implants diverging by up to 60 degrees, but also reduce distortion of the insert. Always begin with the lightest retention force insert (blue), otherwise it can be difficult to remove dentures easily, even when they are retained by only two abutments.

Occasionally, patients may complain of tissue trapping. In this case, you must assess whether this is because of the denture extension or inadequate height of the ISOD abutment. Whilst problems may be similar to those of conventional complete dentures (Chapters 45 and 46), looseness may be because of inadequate torqueing of the abutment or inadequate retention from the female component.

Maintenance

Following rehabilitation, a maintenance programme is key to long-term success. Allowing the tissues to breathe by leaving prostheses out overnight, or for several hours during the day, is recommended.

ISOD abutments should be cleaned with conventional and interdental brushes, and the prostheses themselves should be cleansed in alloy-safe solutions (such as those suitable for cobalt-chrome partial dentures).

At each patient review, in relation to the implants, you should monitor pocket depths. If pockets are bleeding and deepening, despite efforts to improve oral hygiene and remove calculus, then this is indicative of peri-implantitis. This can be confirmed with evidence of crestal bone loss on radiographs. At this stage, it is acceptable to refer the patient to (or recommend that the patient sees) a specialist for treatment of the peri-implantitis.

42 Principles of restoring maxillary defects

Figure 42.1 Principles of restoring maxillary defects

Aramany classification

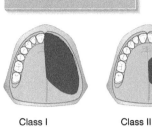 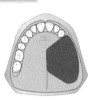 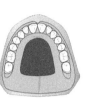   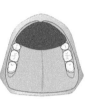

| Class I | Class II | Class III | Class IV | Class V | Class IV |

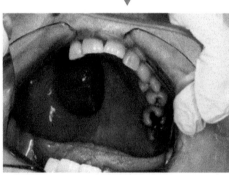

Class II defect requiring rehabilitation

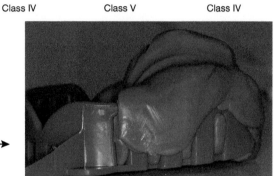

Primary impression of the defect in putty

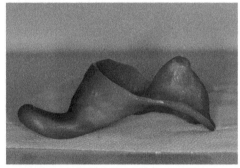

Special tray for alginate, perforated on the fitting surface

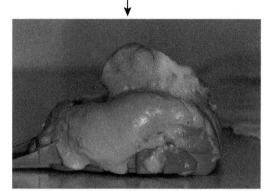

Gauze is then placed across the defect prior to an alginate wash

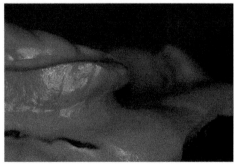

Final wash impression, allowing some engagement of tissue undercut

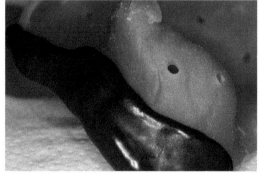

Careful border moulding around the defect and denture periphery

Removable Prosthodontics at a Glance, First Edition. James Field and Claire Storey. © 2020 James Field and Claire Storey. Published 2020 by John Wiley & Sons Ltd.
Companion Website: www.wiley.com/go/field/removable

From time to time, you may encounter patients with maxillary defects. These may be minor, or extensive, developmental or acquired – often the palate, ridges and the teeth are involved, either in isolation or in combination. This chapter aims to describe some of the clinical and design approaches that you may wish to consider when constructing an upper prosthesis for patients with varying Aramany classifications. The prosthesis would be referred to as an *obturator*, because it is closing a congenital or an acquired tissue opening.

Primary impressions

Taking impressions for patients with maxillary defects can be daunting. Primarily, this is because of the appearance of the tissues involved with the defect. Secondarily, you will want to avoid losing impression material into the defect – especially if it is deep or inaccessible. It is well worth taking the time to explore the surrounding anatomy. Palpate the peripheral walls, noting whether the tissue is firm or fibrous. Make a note of the sensation the patient feels when you palpate – and consider whether the tissues can provide support for the prosthesis or aid in retention. It is not necessary to record the full height of the defect. However, recording the full *peripheral* anatomy is important to ensure an adequate oral seal. It is possible to ask the technician to engage a certain amount of undercut within the defect by utilising permanent soft lining material. In the case in Figure 42.1, resistance and retention was gained from the medial, mesial and distal aspects of the defect (palatine bone and anterior nasal spine). Care was taken to avoid heavily engaging the lateral aspect (the alveolar recess of the maxillary sinus) because of its respiratory epithelial lining, which was tender to palpate. In other cases you can look out for bands of scar tissue, which often flex, to allow insertion and improved retention.

Initially, putty is a very useful material to use in a tray. It will largely record the defect and once set it will then help to carry an alginate or silicone wash. It is a good idea to apply gauze across the defect prior to taking a wash impression, to prevent excess material becoming retained.

Major impressions

As always, the extensions of the special tray are critical in obtaining a truly functional impression. Communicate with the technician about where you would like the tray to engage around the defect and how closely. Ensure that the tray is extended properly; we would advise recording the borders of the periphery and critical areas of the defect initially, using greenstick. The wash impression is most often taken in alginate, because this material is most easily removed from undercuts and defects. Remember that only a thin wash is necessary – and leave the impression in situ until it has fully set in order to facilitate complete removal.

Framework designs

Whilst it is a good idea to remember the standard design principles for partial prostheses, there are some principles that

necessarily differ. There is little doubt in these cases that a rigid and full coverage major connector is most useful.

We will discuss a number of design considerations for the various defect configurations (Figure 42.1) below:
• *Class I – Full unilateral defect to the midline.* Consider placing occlusal rests on the most medial and distal surfaces. Placing double rests can prevent wedging forces because of the large torqueing effect of the poorly supported saddle. Extending up to the palatal surfaces can maximise bracing and stability. With full coverage designs, ensuring adequate oral hygiene is paramount.
• *Class II – A single unilateral defect not involving the premaxilla.* Indirect retention is important here and this can be obtained by resting on the canine that is furthest away from the defect. A tripod design with double rests on the posterior teeth and engagement of the palatal surfaces will maximise bracing and stability. Consider smaller occlusal tables with fewer posterior teeth.
• *Class III – A midline defect of the hard palate.* Aside from the absence of prosthetic saddles, the design approach is largely similar to many Kennedy Class III presentations. A quadratic clasping approach is recommended in the absence of any palatal support.
• *Class IV – A single unilateral posterior and premaxillary defect.* This presentation is challenging because of the presence of a single line of teeth. Ensuring correct extensions is critical. Consider using multiple clasps with mesial and distal rests or placing indirect restorations with milled shoulders, guide planes and even channels or pins. Once again, a reduced occlusal table will be helpful.
• *Class V – A bilateral posterior defect.* Again, indirect retention is important here, given the forced symmetry of the clasping axis. This may involve coverage of the palatal surfaces. An RPI (rest, plate, I-bar clasp) approach can be considered to reduce torque on the abutment teeth. For both this and class IV presentations, you might consider a swing lock design if the abutment teeth were periodontally sound, well-supported and there was sufficient sulcus depth.
• *Class VI – A single anterior bilateral defect.* This is quite a rare presentation and usually presents because of trauma or congenital conditions. This is essentially managed as a Kennedy Class IV design, maximising indirect retention. In this case, a lack of anterior soft tissue support also means that a quadratic clasping design is preferred.

Obturator bungs

The bung is the portion of the obturator that engages the defect. Two main types exist. *Extended hollow bulbs* engage more of the defect and are therefore better supported. Rigidity means that problems with leakage are common, although the hollow nature of the bulb improves speech resonance and reduces the weight. The alternative is an *open top with a flexible bung* – this design is able to atraumatically engage undercuts and provide an excellent seal. The drawback of this design is the fact that the permanent soft liner material will perish more quickly and adjustments to the fitting surface can be difficult.

43 Tissue conditioners, liners and re-basing

Figure 43.1 Tissue conditioners, liners and rebasing

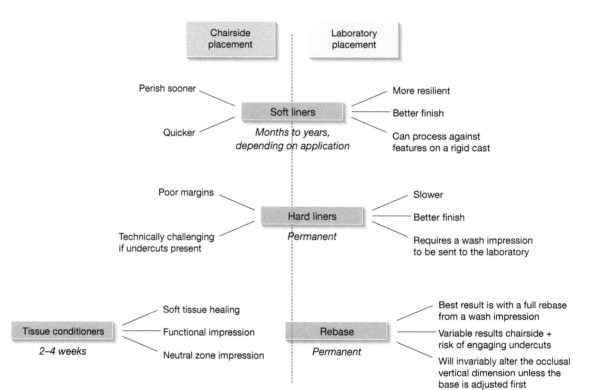

Chairside placement | Laboratory placement

Soft liners — *Months to years, depending on application*
- Perish sooner
- Quicker
- More resilient
- Better finish
- Can process against features on a rigid cast

Hard liners — *Permanent*
- Poor margins
- Technically challenging if undercuts present
- Slower
- Better finish
- Requires a wash impression to be sent to the laboratory

Tissue conditioners — *2–4 weeks*
- Soft tissue healing
- Functional impression
- Neutral zone impression

Rebase — *Permanent*
- Best result is with a full rebase from a wash impression
- Variable results chairside + risk of engaging undercuts
- Will invariably alter the occlusal vertical dimension unless the base is adjusted first

An example of a laboratory placed soft liner. Often a well extended lower complete impression will engage minor undercuts around the lingual shelf. Engaging with a soft liner rather than under-extending or adjusting the base can help to maintain a border seal and reduce lingual trauma

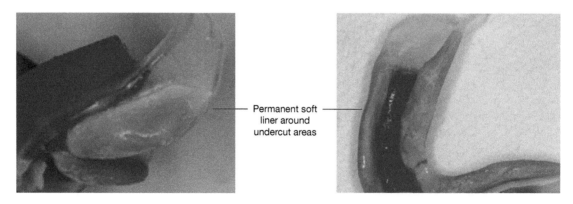

Permanent soft liner around undercut areas

From time to time, it may be necessary for you to adjust and augment a finished denture base significantly. This may be for the following reasons:
- Changes in ridge anatomy
- Over- or underextension into the functional sulcus
- Relief over an area of trauma, surgery or a superficial nerve
- Alterations to the occlusal vertical dimension
- Alterations to avoid fabrication of a totally new prosthesis

When augmenting the denture base, the materials and methods that you use will be dependent on a number of factors (outlined in Figure 43.1). These include:
- Junctions and marginal finish
- Accuracy
- Material availability, technique and chairside time
- Expected resilience and longevity of the addition
- Laboratory requirements

The most significant challenge when relining or rebasing, regardless of where the processing will occur (at the chairside or in the laboratory), is the ability to control the denture during the moulding stage. Polished denture surfaces and the absence of a handle make it difficult to ensure stability and correct seating prior to tissue manipulation. The only exception to this is the use of a *tissue conditioner*.

Tissue conditioners

Tissue conditioners can remain in situ for 2–4 weeks, depending on the specific product – and because of the high volume of plasticiser present in the material, the tissue conditioner continues to be moulded in function whilst the patient uses the prosthesis. This is useful for obtaining functional border extensions in difficult cases, such as in patients being rehabilitated after oncology treatment or after suffering a stroke. Tissue conditioners are also extremely useful for temporary re-lines around areas of trauma or recent surgery, or for neutral zone impressions. Tissue conditioners tend to be coloured white as a reminder of their temporary nature. However, some soft lining systems allow you to alter the mixing ratio to determine how resilient and how *temporary* you would like the material to be. In these cases, the colour is consistent regardless of the application. Tissue conditioners are typically mixed from a polymer powder (usually polyethyl methacrylate, or PEMA) and a plasticiser and monomer liquid. Regardless of the product used, the prosthesis should be physically and chemically cleaned prior to application. Most soft liner products include an 'adhesive' that actually just cleans the surface prior to application – this tends to be a ketone-based solvent.

Soft liners

Soft liners (sometimes known as resilient liners) can be semipermanent or permanent. Chairside applied liners tend to be semipermanent in nature and may last months or even years depending on their mode of use and area of application. They can be categorised as silicone elastomers or plasticised acrylic resins. The silicone-based materials are more resistant to leaching their plasticisers. They are commonly used where undercuts (either occurring naturally or post-surgery) need to be engaged comfortably; this may have been trialled first with a tissue conditioner. Soft liners can also distribute loads more comfortably over localised painful areas, although we would urge against prescribing a full-coverage soft liner where the patient claims it makes the denture(s) more comfortable. This seems a logical thing to do, but practically this prevents occlusal forces being distributed evenly across the full denture-bearing area. Paradoxically, this causes rocking, tipping, aberrant occlusal contacts and areas of localised pain.

Soft liners placed at the chairside may require trimming and finishing to make the interface with the acrylic as seamless as possible. Specific silicone burs should be used for this purpose. Where a longer term need for the soft liner exists such as in oncology or cleft defects, then a more resilient, laboratory-provided soft liner should be considered at the time of prosthesis fabrication.

Degradation

Over the relatively short life of the tissue conditioner, plasticiser will leach from the material leading to a loss of surface integrity and a rough surface. This can inflame the denture-bearing area and encourage a reservoir of bacteria and fungi to reside against the tissues. Chairside soft liner materials are more resilient than tissue conditioners, but will ultimately suffer the same fate. Antifungal and bacterial agents may be present in the materials to counteract the growing microbial reservoir, but by the time this becomes a problem, the prosthesis should have been definitively modified or replaced. Surface degradation can also cause these materials to peel away from the underlying prosthesis; this can also happen if the material becomes degraded or if vigorous hygiene techniques are used. Cleaning is recommended with a soft brush, sponge or the patient's fingertips under lukewarm water with liquid soap.

Re-basing

Re-basing is the term given to replacing the entire intaglio denture surface and borders in hard acrylic whilst preserving the tooth arrangement and other polished surfaces. A chairside re-base should be avoided because autopolymerising acrylic is not as stable in the longer term and carries with it a risk of curing into undercuts at the chairside. It is difficult to handle, is exothermic in large quantities and carries with it considerable room for errors. Hard re-line of partial dentures should also be approached with considerable caution, especially where multiple short spans are present, with drifted and tilted teeth, and bony undercuts. Instead, a silicone impression and laboratory re-base is recommended.

For any hard re-line or re-base procedure at the chairside, undercuts should be blocked out using wax, temporary inlay material or silicone. The prosthesis should be removed and reinserted as it goes through its exothermic reaction to ensure it is able to be removed and reinserted with ease along a single path of insertion. Excess should be removed chairside with an acrylic bur and the prosthesis polished to ensure it is cleansable and comfortable.

44 Maintaining adequate oral hygiene

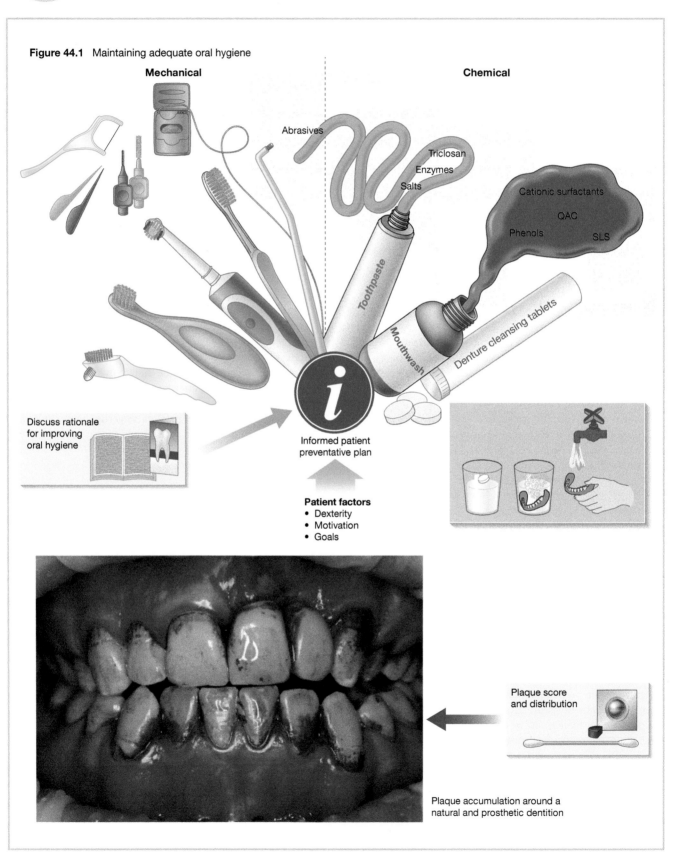

Figure 44.1 Maintaining adequate oral hygiene

Mechanical

Chemical

Abrasives

Triclosan
Enzymes
Salts

Cationic surfactants

QAC

Phenols

SLS

Toothpaste

Mouthwash

Denture cleansing tablets

Discuss rationale for improving oral hygiene

Informed patient preventative plan

Patient factors
- Dexterity
- Motivation
- Goals

Plaque score and distribution

Plaque accumulation around a natural and prosthetic dentition

Removable Prosthodontics at a Glance, First Edition. James Field and Claire Storey. © 2020 James Field and Claire Storey. Published 2020 by John Wiley & Sons Ltd.
Companion Website: www.wiley.com/go/field/removable

aintaining adequate oral hygiene is a shared responsibility between clinician and patient. As dental professionals we are expected (either individually or as a team) to inform the patient of:

- The rationale for good oral hygiene
- Their current level of oral hygiene
- Patient-specific optimal methods
- Individual progress in maintaining adequate oral hygiene

Instigating and maintaining behaviour change can be time consuming – and it is important for the patient to understand that they have very much an active role. If the patient does not believe, or understand, the need for adequate plaque control then they are unlikely to build suitable habits into their daily routines. We can help the patient on their journey by removing calculus and charting the location of plaque. A full mouth prophylaxis can also help to motivate the patient.

The impact of partial prostheses

Patients must understand the extra burden that removable prostheses place on maintaining adequate plaque control. It is for this reason that adequate oral hygiene efforts should be demonstrated by the patient before a prosthesis is provided. Once the prosthesis is in place, the patient will face the challenge of greater food debris accumulation, greater plaque accumulation and the need to satisfactorily clean the dental tissues *and* the prosthesis itself. This is no small task, and once a partial prosthesis is fitted, part of the review process should include an assessment of the patient's ability to keep it clean.

The patient should also understand that there are significant risks to wearing a prosthesis continually. The main risk is that of root caries, as plaque and other food debris are held against exposed root surfaces for long periods of time. Without adequate and timely management, a biofilm will develop and mature, encouraging an anaerobic environment and promoting bacterial growth that is more resistant to removal by conventional means and that is increasingly pathogenic.

Patients should be encouraged to leave their prosthesis out overnight – failing this, for several hours during the day. This allows intraoral surfaces to be cleansed by saliva and the tongue, and for the prosthesis to be mechanically cleaned, followed by immersion in a suitable cleaning solution.

Complicating factors

It is important for us to be able to identify elements of prosthetic design that, combined with the patient's social and medical history, may increase the risks of plaque accumulation and caries. There is little doubt that ensuring a prosthesis sits at least 3 mm from the gingival margins is a useful approach to reduce food and plaque accumulation against the hard tissues; however, acrylic resin will deteriorate over time, especially as

surface imperfections begin to develop. Acrylic resin is already a relatively porous material on a microscopic level, which is why storing the prosthesis in a solution is such an important part of the hygiene protocol. Cobalt-chrome materials and ceramics are much more resistant to plaque accumulation, although the design of major connectors will impact significantly on oral hygiene, and these are discussed in Chapter 31.

Patient factors that may increase the risk of plaque accumulation and caries further include:

- Poor manual dexterity
- Lack of suitable oral hygiene equipment
- Poor understanding of hygiene procedures
- Dietary risk factors
- Xerostomia
- Systemic disease states such as diabetes
- Nicotine use and smoking

The patient should be made aware of these risks, when present, and suitable preventive measures put into place. This may include liaising with the patient's general medical practitioner, certainly in relation to diabetic control, xerostomia because of polypharmacy and smoking cessation. In the dentate patient, oral hygiene should be undertaken on a bi-daily basis including mechanical and chemical plaque control. It is not within the scope of this chapter to discuss this further but Figure 44.1 highlights the important techniques and materials.

Cleaning partial and complete prostheses

Even a highly polished acrylic denture is plaque retentive and so this should first be cleaned mechanically with liquid soap over a water-filled sink. This ensures that the prosthesis does not fracture if dropped. Toothpastes are effective in removing bacteria but not fungal colonisation, and *abrasive* toothpastes (such as whitening pastes) should be avoided on acrylic because this will create a more plaque-retentive surface. If there is no metal base on the denture then up to 6% hypochlorite may be used for 20 minutes prior to storage in water. This gives excellent antimicrobial results. Care must be taken with cobalt-chrome-based dentures, because hypochlorite will cause corrosion and pitting, and certain acidic cleansers will cause a black oxide layer to form on the prosthesis. Recent reviews have shown that specialist denture cleanser tablets give a good combination of microbial efficacy and reasonable material compatibility.

Fixed prostheses

Communication with the laboratory is essential to produce a fixed prosthesis that favours patient self-care and maintenance. Providing your technician with an interdental brush can help to create adequate embrasure spaces for cleansing and to design contact against abutment teeth that will prevent food impaction, gum stripping and abutment disease.

Troubleshooting loose or painful dentures

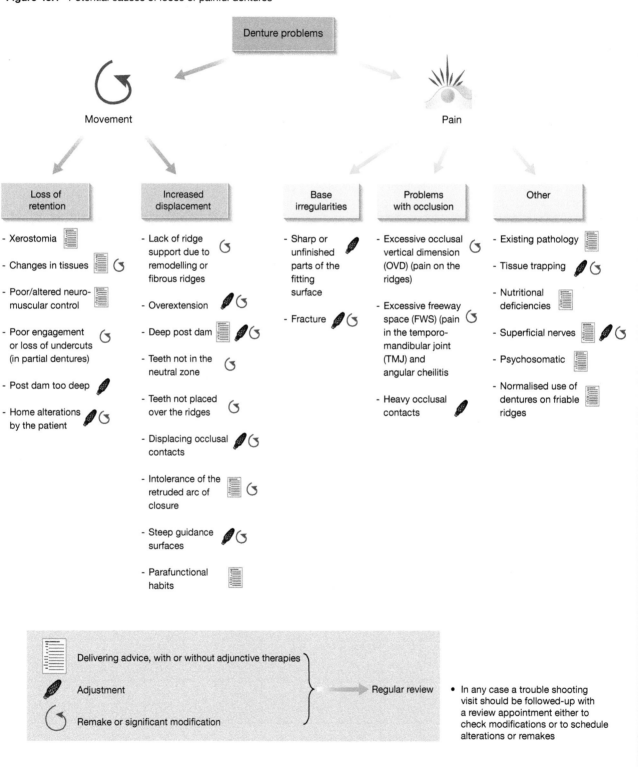

Figure 45.1 Potential causes of loose or painful dentures

Removable Prosthodontics at a Glance, First Edition. James Field and Claire Storey. © 2020 James Field and Claire Storey. Published 2020 by John Wiley & Sons Ltd.
Companion Website: www.wiley.com/go/field/removable

Regardless of the stages of denture construction or review, it is important to be able to troubleshoot the causes of instability and pain. We most commonly see these problems either soon after dentures are fitted or when patients present to us wanting new dentures to be made – but they can also present *during* construction. There are a number of ways to pre-empt these problems and reduce the number of complications. At all stages, ensure that your patient is forewarned about potential complications, including pain under the dentures and instability. Forewarned is forearmed – and if you have already discussed potential problems with your patient, then they are less likely to be surprised when they occur. This helps to maintain a trusting relationship and shows that you are mindful of complications, and that you are in control of managing them. However, it can also be incredibly frustrating when you are unable to find a direct cause, or indeed a suitable solution, to denture pain. I find that following a logical and systematic approach means that you are unlikely to miss out any less-obvious causes. The flow diagrams in Figure 45.1 can help to guide you through this troubleshooting process.

Loss of retention and displacement

Looseness or mobility of dentures is caused, primarily, by both a loss of retention and an increase in displacement forces.

Loss of retention

One of the benefits of employing a permanent base for the jaw relation stage and beyond is that you are able to test the *actual* retention and stability of the prosthesis prior to fitting. Otherwise, it can always be quite tense at the fit stage, when you have been working, thus far, with a temporary base – border extension inaccuracies may not be apparent during construction. Some clinicians tell patients at the fit stage that they will need to wait for their dentures to 'bed in'. This is by no means a panacea for ill-fitting dentures, although there is *some* truth in this instruction – often, when old dentures are removed and new ones fitted straight away, a degree of soft tissue recoil is required in order to allow close adaptation of the new denture base. This is especially true if the working impression has taken a relatively long time to make. Normally, tissue recoil happens within 10–20 minutes – and as mentioned above, it is always helpful to pre-empt these particular nuances with the patient.

Other possible causes of lack of retention and instability include:
- Xerostomia
- Changes in tissue fluid (in patients who take steroids periodically)
- A lack of appreciation of the need for muscular control
- For partial dentures, lack of a defined path of insertion (meaning that multiple adjustments have likely been made in order to fit the prosthesis, with resulting dead spaces and poor adaptation to abutment teeth)

Increased displacement

An increase in displacement can be observed in the following cases:
- Ridge changes because of remodelling following extractions
- Overextension in sulcal depth and width

- An excessively deep post dam
- Failure to place teeth within the neutral zone
- Failure to place teeth directly over the ridges
- Displacing occlusal contacts
- An intolerance of a shift to a more retruded arc of closure
- Lack of freedom in intercuspal position (steep guiding surfaces)
- Lack of support from the edentulous ridge(s)
- Pain avoidance mechanisms and parafunctional habits

Pain underneath denture bases

When we hear patients reporting pain from the fitting surface of a denture, often the first instinct is to pick up a hand piece and make some adjustments. I would suggest that this course of action should be one of the *last* things that you do – there is no going back from this intervention and it sets up a futile cycle of adjustments. However, minor adjustments to surface *finish* will not affect the fit and adaptation of the denture – as soon as you receive the permanent base back from the technician, it is a good idea to run your gloved fingers over the fitting surface and remove any obviously sharp lips, bumps and rough areas with a polishing bur.

By far the most common cause for pain over the ridges is incorrect, premature or heavy occlusal contacts. Checking contacts in the intercuspal position with articulating paper should form a routine part of your troubleshooting process, even if you have identified another obvious case. If frank ulceration is present, then I would recommend that the patient leaves their denture out until this has resolved. It is possible to make some adjustments at the same appointment but be wary of adjusting the denture base *so* much that the pain no longer presents – it is likely in this case that you have overadjusted the denture base, which may result in instability, food trapping, or pain elsewhere on the ridge. In the absence of any pathology, it is a good idea to palpate the ridge with a gloved finger. Sometimes patients report pain over the ridge when there is no obvious cause – and this can be a frustrating presentation. Paradoxically, patients who have not been wearing dentures for a while (or who have been coping with ill-fitting dentures) often report pain when they begin to use dentures effectively again, especially if they are more stable. It is important to reassure this group of patients and to pre-empt the problem by offering eating advice – softer and smaller food choices for the first few weeks, and chewing at the back of the mouth, on both sides. Occasionally during denture assessment, patients present with pain on the ridge even with gentle loading – in these cases, it may be necessary to consider relief over the crest of the ridge at the construction stage. Ultimately, you may wish to refer these patients for a specialist opinion.

Other causes of pain

Other common causes of pain include:
- Heel clash of the denture bases causing tissue trapping (check with articulating paper between the heels)
- Nutritional deficiencies (B_{12}, folate) that predispose to ulceration or symptoms of oral dysaesthesia

46 Gagging, other difficulties and making a referral

Figure 46.1 Gagging, and speech

Gagging

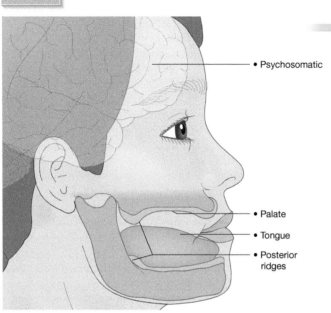

- Psychosomatic
- Palate
- Tongue
- Posterior ridges

- Explore with the patient the history of their gag reflex
- Palpate the full denture bearing area in order to better understand the potential trigger zones and what the patient currently tolerates

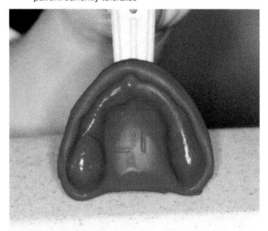

Consider a training impression or plate – but counsel the patient on how to use it effectively (see text)

Speech 9/12

- Can take up to 9 months to acclimatise
- Especially if tooth positions have changed
- Read aloud each day in order to improve control

Palatal tongue contact patterns

Consider patterns of tongue contact if particular phonetics are challenging for the patient

Contact area

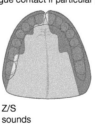 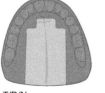 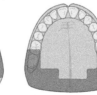 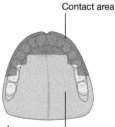

| T/D/N sounds | Z/S sounds | Sh sounds | K/G sounds | L sounds | Non-contact area |

Consider freeway space if 's' sounds are whistling or hollow
- Very hollow suggests excessive freeway space (FWS)
- Whistling or sharp 's' sounds suggests restricted FWS

Removable Prosthodontics at a Glance, First Edition. James Field and Claire Storey. © 2020 James Field and Claire Storey. Published 2020 by John Wiley & Sons Ltd.
Companion Website: www.wiley.com/go/field/removable

From time to time you may encounter particularly challenging presentations. This chapter considers how to deal with a severe gag reflex, hyperactive tongue and lips, and speech problems. Aspects of the referral process are covered in Appendix 3.

Managing the gagging patient

I would consider a severe gag reflex to be one of the most challenging situations facing prosthodontists. It is recognised that the acceptance of dentures in gagging patients will improve with continued and persistent use. However, the aetiology is considered to be multifactorial, and many psychologists recognise that the gag reflex is classically conditioned. This means that patients can present with significant and deeply embedded fear-related components. In its milder forms of presentation, the gag reflex can simply be an anxious response to denture instability. Constructing a properly extended and stable prosthesis is often all that is needed – and the patient should be reassured as such. Occasionally a more structured approach is needed and this is described below.

Functional analysis and patient control

Functional analysis is a well-established approach for supporting patients through difficult treatments. This comprises:
- Building a trusting and relaxed relationship
- A careful history of specific trigger factors
- Investigation of the patient's concerns and stressors
- A direct observation of the problem
- Continual clinical observation during procedures

One of overarching principles for the treatment of patients who gag is *allowing the patient to feel that they are in control*. This does not mean, however, that dentures should be removed from the mouth as soon as a gag reflex is elicited. On the contrary, immediate removal is a behaviour which will perpetuate the gag reflex, regardless of how hard patients try and persevere. The principle is to give the patient the tools to overcome any anxieties they might hold about wearing a prosthesis.

A simple primary impression in compound (which is robust and cleansable) can be taken home and used as an acclimatisation tray. It *must* have a handle and be fully extended (Figure 46.1). Patients should spend regular time each day in a calm and stress-free environment. They should attempt to retain the impression as long as possible, with careful and controlled breathing. When they begin to gag, they should sit calmly and focus on their breathing – the impression should *not* be removed each time the urge arrives – yet the patient themselves must be in control. With this approach, even before completion of new dentures, the patient is often able to tolerate the necessary clinical stages. A similar approach can be adopted with an acrylic training plate, or a series of training plates – however, in my experience, it is easier and more effective to simply provide a full arch impression that comprehensively covers the denture-bearing area and the full depth of the sulci.

On occasion, we are unable to overcome patients' pathological reflexes and it may be necessary to consider adjuncts such as acupuncture or referring the patient (via their general medical practitioner) to a clinical psychologist. In my experience, this only applies to a minority of patients. The vast majority should be reassured in a calm and confident manner, and given the space and opportunity to acclimatise themselves to wearing a full-coverage prosthesis.

Tongue spread and lip activity

Lateral spread or hyperactivity of the tongue or lower lip can be incredibly frustrating to manage. In these cases, it is important to explain to the patient what is happening and how they can try and help. Like any muscle, the tongue will lose tone if it is not in continual use. Patients who do not currently wear lower prostheses routinely will need to re-acclimatise – and this often involves a bit of homework. It is possible to give patients a series of simple exercises that can allow them to regain some muscular awareness and control. These are described below and should be demonstrated to the patient first, with the recommendation that they are carried out in front of a mirror:
- Slide the thumb along the upper ridge from tuberosity to tuberosity whilst keeping the tongue relaxed, without allowing the tongue to touch the thumb, especially posteriorly
- Slide the index finger along the lower ridge whilst the tongue slides as far back as possible and away from the index finger
- Consciously relax the lower lip to allow palpation of the anterior crest of the ridge with an index finger
- Look carefully at the tongue in a mirror and do not let it escape the mouth or cross over the vermillion border of the lower lip whilst resting

Speech problems

Most patients will adapt quickly to speaking with their new prosthesis, assuming that there have not been significant changes to the incisal relationship or palatal contour. Nonetheless this can take up to 9 months, or even longer in some cases. Alteration to speech can be a cause of great concern to your patients – and once again this needs a sympathetic and systematic approach. I tend to find that prescribing adequate *speaking* space at the prescription stage (see Chapter 23) avoids subsequent problems. The evidence suggests that, in the first instance, patients should be encouraged to read out loud for at least an hour each day. This can improve both speech and masticatory function.

However, sometimes patients are more concerned about subtle alterations to their speech. Often this will relate to how the tongue is interacting with the denture base palatally – this can be checked with a dusting of pressure relief cream onto the polished surface palatally. Tongue contact will be directly visible – this should appear largely in line with the patterns in Figure 46.1. It is possible to add carding wax diagnostically onto existing dentures in order to alter the relationship to the tongue. This contour can then be copied by the technician.

Referral process

Appendix 3 details what information should be included in a referral letter.

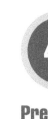

47 Summary of procedural stages

Prescribing the placement of teeth and recording jaw relations

- Check the prescription blocks
  - Retention and fit
  - This is often easier with permanent bases
  - Any changes you make to temporary bases will be lost during final processing
- Modify lip support and incisal level on the upper rim
  - Alma gauge to compare with the previous denture
  - Fox's plane guide to assess incisal plane and alar–tragal plane
  - Pare out waxwork palatally to make room for tongue
- Mark centre lines, canine lines and smile line
  - Decide on reference point for centre line
  - Canine tips in line with alar of nose and inner canthus of eye
- Check buccal corridors
  - 2–3 mm of buccal space with a wide smile
  - Bevel the wax block on a hot plate to create space
- Adjust lower rim to occlude evenly with upper
  - Don't worry about occlusal vertical dimension yet
  - Achieve even contact first
  - Use a wax plate to ensure flat occlusal planes
- Modify lower rim to maximise stability and speech
  - Consider neutral zone
  - Pare out excess wax lingually to create tongue space
  - Check speaking space
- Adjust occlusal vertical dimension
  - Based on speaking space and appearance
  - Whistling sounds suggest restricted space
  - Hollow sounds suggest excessive space
- Re-confirm even contact in retruded arc of closure
  - Take care to identify and avoid heel clash
- Mark with buccal check marks and cut opposing notches bilaterally
  - Deep square notches down to the denture base
- Close passively and register with silicone
  - Gently hold the patient in the intended intercuspal position whilst syringing silicone registration paste into the opposing notches
- Check for heel clash
  - If present, adjust and re-register
- Check for reproducibility after disassembly
  - Disassemble and reassemble prior to disinfection
- Select mould and shade
- Copy old tooth set-up or arrangement, in alginate, if needed
- Write laboratory prescription and package disinfected records carefully

Partial denture design

- Ensure accurate and contemporaneous periodontal assessment
  - 6-point pocket chart or Basic Periodontal Examination as a minimum
  - Plaque and bleeding scores
  - Mobility scores
  - Radiographs of potential abutment teeth
- Obtain accurate study models
  - Well-extended trays
  - Pre-loading of difficult areas
  - Ensure material is supported by the tray
- Accurately articulate
  - Employ registration blocks where tripod contacts are not possible
  - Detail expected tooth contacts to laboratory
- Study each cast making notes of:
  - Ridge undercuts
  - Dead spaces
  - Guide planes
  - Teeth unable to support a prosthesis
  - Teeth of poor prognosis and anticipated loss
- Prescribe saddles
  - Ensure full ridge coverage
  - Saddles do not necessarily indicate the replacement of teeth
- Rests
  - Occlusal support at each saddle junction
  - Consider if tooth can support a rest axially
  - Tooth preparation often needed
  - Check articulation for occlusal space
  - Rounded to allow movement in function
  - Consider onlay or shoulder elements
- Clasps
  - Direct retentive elements
  - Must be accompanied by a rest
  - Consider an asymmetrical and anterioposteriorly discrepant clasping axis
  - Consider how the clasp assembly connects to the major connector, and the robustness of the design
- Indirect retention
  - Consider rest or saddle elements far away from the clasping axis, that will prevent tipping
- Bracing
  - Consider major connector extension over ridges and into palate
  - Consider proximal plates
- Reciprocation
  - Reciprocate clasp arms with a reciprocating arm, a ring clasp, or the major connector itself
  - Consider how elements connect together
  - Consider the robustness of the design
- Major connector
  - Consider rigidity, cleansability, mucosal coverage, bracing, cohesion/adhesion
  - Ensure connectors and the design are as simple as possible
- Survey
  - Mark survey lines for the path of natural displacement and the intended path of insertion (if different)
  - Tilt the casts to reduce dead spaces and engage guide planes
  - Consider augmenting teeth with flowable composite if undercut is required

Removable Prosthodontics at a Glance, First Edition. James Field and Claire Storey. © 2020 James Field and Claire Storey. Published 2020 by John Wiley & Sons Ltd.
Companion Website: www.wiley.com/go/field/removable

- Consider replacing existing crowns if rest seats or other supportive elements need to be prepared
- Clearly communicate the design, including intended paths of insertion, to the laboratory

Partial denture provision
- Patient assessment (see Appendix 2)
  - Including discussion of patient expectations
- Obtain accurate study models
  - Well-extended trays
  - Pre-loading of difficult areas
  - Ensure material is supported by the tray
- Accurately articulate
  - Employ registration blocks where tripod contacts are not possible
- Denture design
  - Still important for acrylic dentures
  - Define a path of insertion
  - Prescribe cast elements where necessary
- Obtain special trays
  - Define impression material to be used
  - Request tissue stops if needed
- Tooth modifications
  - Where necessary
  - Rest seats
  - Guide planes
  - Place or replace extra-coronal restorations
- Functional impressions
  - Ensure adequate tray adjustment
  - Do not overfill the tray
  - Ensure fully seated with functional border moulding
- Framework try-in
  - Check design
  - Check path of insertion
  - Seat using rest elements only
  - Check occlusion
- Recording jaw relations and prescribing tooth positions
  - Maintain existing natural tooth contacts or
  - Choose a new occlusal vertical dimension
  - Record the relationship passively
  - Record shade and mould
- Try-in
  - Check fit and stability
  - Check occlusion
  - Check aesthetics and speech
- Fit
- Review

Complete denture provision
- Patient assessment (see Appendix 1)
  - Including discussion of patient expectations
- Obtain accurate primary impressions
  - Ensure full coverage of the denture-bearing area
  - Consider copying dentures in putty if largely correct or easily extended
- Obtain special trays
  - Define impression material to be used
  - Request tissue stops if needed
- Functional impressions
  - Ensure adequate tray adjustment

- Do not overfill the tray
- Ensure fully seated with functional border moulding
- Recording jaw relations and prescribing tooth positions
  - Upper block for aesthetics
  - Lower block for stability
  - Record the relationship passively
  - Check for heel clash
  - Record shade and mould
- Try-in
  - Check fit and stability
  - Check occlusion
  - Check aesthetics and speech
- Fit
- Review

Modified copy denture provision
- Patient assessment (see Appendix 1)
  - Discuss patient expectations
  - Confirm denture extensions are largely correct
- Obtain accurate copies of the denture(s)
  - Use metal copy boxes
  - Ensure copies are free from large voids and other defects
- Recording jaw relations and prescribing tooth positions
  - Replica dentures should be largely correct
  - Check upper block for aesthetics
  - Check lower block for stability
  - Record the relationship passively
  - Check for heel clash
  - Record shade
- Try-in
  - Check fit and stability
  - Check occlusion
  - Check aesthetics and speech
  - Remove undercuts from fitting surface of acrylic base
  - Functional impression – closed mouth, one arch at a time
  - Do not overfill the tray
  - Functional border moulding
- Fit
- Review

Implant-supported mandibular overdenture provision
- Patient assessment (see Appendix 1)
  - Discuss patient expectations
  - Determine attachment system
  - Determine abutment heights
  - Order necessary components
- Obtain accurate primary impressions
  - Ensure full coverage of the denture-bearing area
- Obtain special trays
  - Specify open or closed tray
  - If closed tray, ensure laboratory prescribe relief over the intended implant abutments
  - Define impression material to be used
  - Request tissue stops if needed
- Functional impressions
  - Ensure adequate tray adjustment
  - Attach abutments and impression copings
  - Use an accurate silicone or polyether material
  - Ensure fully seated with functional border moulding

- Attach laboratory analogues into the impression copings within the impression
  - Request a permanent base
- Recording jaw relations and prescribing tooth positions
  - Upper block for aesthetics
  - Lower block for stability (less so if retained well on the permanent base)
  - Record the relationship passively
  - Check for heel clash
  - Record shade and mould

- Try-in
  - Check fit and stability
  - Check occlusion
  - Check aesthetics and speech
- Fit
  - Activate implant attachment system if necessary
  - Ensure patient can insert and remove
  - Discuss implant health and maintenance
- Review

Appendices

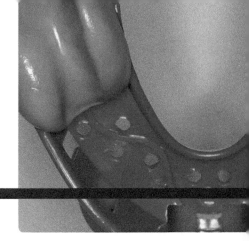

Appendix 1: Complete denture assessment proforma

Appendix 1

Department of Restorative Dentistry
Complete Denture Assessment Clinic

Clinician _____ Date _____

☐ Medical History checked ☐ *complicated*

☐ Gender ☐ Age

☐ Place patient label here

Why does the patient want new dentures?

☐ Loose upper denture ☐ *at rest* ☐ *when eating*

☐ Loose lower denture ☐ *at rest* ☐ *when eating*

☐ Denture pain ☐ *upper* ☐ *lower* **Other details**

☐ Difficulty chewing ☐ *worse recently* ☐ Acrylic

☐ Difficulty speaking ☐ *worse recently* ☐ Co-Cr

☐ Nausea ☐ *at rest* ☐ *eating* ☐ *speaking* ☐ Age of denture (years)

☐ Intolerance ☐ *immediate (within 5 seconds)* ☐ Total years edentulous

☐ Worn denture(s) ☐ *local* ☐ *generalised* ☐ Total number of sets

☐ Poor appearance _____

Extra-oral examination Left (L) Right (R) or Bilateral (B) No positive findings ☐

☐ TMJ ☐ *Click* ☐ *Pain* ☐ *Lock* ☐ *Crepitus*

☐ Palpable nodes

☐ Muscle pain ☐ *Masseter* ☐ *Temporalis* ☐ *SCM* ☐ *Other* _____

☐ Glands ☐ *Currently suffering from known systemic illness*

Clinical examination

Intra-oral access ☐ *good* ☐ *restricted* _____

Tongue ☐ *normal* ☐ *lateral spread* ☐ *hyperactive*

Gag reflex ☐ *tongue* ☐ *palate*

Ulceration ☐ _____

Candidosis ☐

Angular cheilitis ☐

Dry mouth ☐

Tori ☐ *palate* ☐ *lower lingual* ☐ *other* _____

Retained roots ☐ *sound* ☐ *carious*

Suspicious lesion ☐

Other information

Tongue   FOM

Sulcus   Palate

Removable Prosthodontics at a Glance, First Edition. James Field and Claire Storey. © 2020 James Field and Claire Storey. Published 2020 by John Wiley & Sons Ltd.
Companion Website: www.wiley.com/go/field/removable

Ridge assessment

Upper ridge	☐ well-formed	☐ atrophic	☐ rounded	☐ flat ☐ knife-edge	☐ fibrous	☐ undercut
Lower ridge	☐ well-formed	☐ atrophic	☐ rounded	☐ flat ☐ knife-edge	☐ fibrous	
Upper frenae	☐ low/absent	☐ high				
Lower frenae	☐ low/absent	☐ high				

Upper stability and retention:				**Lower stability and retention:**			
Stability	☐ good	☐ fair	☐ poor	Stability	☐ good	☐ fair	☐ poor
Retention	☐ good	☐ fair	☐ poor	Retention	☐ good	☐ fair	☐ poor

Upper denture extensions:				**Lower denture extensions:**			
Labial	☐ correct	☐ under	☐ over	Labial	☐ correct	☐ under	☐ over
Buccal	☐ correct	☐ under	☐ over	Buccal	☐ correct	☐ under	☐ over
Posterior	☐ correct	☐ under	☐ over	Posterior	☐ correct	☐ under	☐ over
Tuberosities	☐ correct	☐ under	☐ over	Lingual	☐ correct	☐ under	☐ over

Aesthetics:				**Occlusion:**			
Acceptable	☐ yes	☐ no	☐	Heavy contacts	☐ no	☐ yes _____	
Lip support	☐ good	☐ high	☐ low	Stable ICP	☐ yes	☐ no	
Incisal plane	☐ correct	☐ incorrect	☐	ICP=RAC	☐ yes	☐ no	
Buccal space	☐ present	☐ absent	☐	FWS	☐ mm		
Mould/shade	☐ accept	☐ change		Speaking space	☐ sufficient	☐ restricted	

Special investigations and other information:

Diagnosis:

Communication:

Explained plan ☐

Patient expectations ☐ reasonable ☐ high

Prognosis for success ☐ guarded ☐ good

Treatment plan in relation to:

Impression surface:

Occlusal surface:

Aesthetics:

Techniques suggested:

Neutral zone ☐

Muco-compressive ☐

Muco-static ☐

Signed: _____ Date: _____

Appendix 2: Restorative assessment proforma

Department of Restorative Dentistry
Adult Assessment Form

Clinician _____ Date _____

☐ Medical History checked   Gender   M : F   Age

Relevant medical history

☐ Place patient label here

Dental history

Last attendance: _____   ☐ Sporadic

☐ Regular attender   ☐ Previous bad experience

☐ Nervous/anxious   ☐ Currently in pain

Principal presenting complaint(s), relevant history and pain history (SOCRATES):

Secondary complaint(s) and relevant history

Patient expectations of treatment and outcome:

Other relevant dental history:

Social history
Occupation _____

☐ Barriers to attendance   ☐ Work   ☐ Dependents   ☐ Other _____

☐ Smoker   ☐ Previous   ☐ Current _____ No/day   ☐ SCA given   ☐ Referral offered

☐ Consumes alcohol   ☐ Units/week and type _____

☐ Recreational drug use

Current preventive regime

☐ Brushing   ☐ Manual   ☐ Electric   ☐ Ultrasonic _____ Times per day

☐ Interdental   ☐ Floss   ☐ Brushes   ☐ Sticks   ☐ Other _____   ☐ Regularly

☐ Mouthwash   ☐ Fluoride   ☐ CHX   ☐ Other _____

☐ Toothpaste   ☐ Fluoride   ☐ Sensitive   ☐ Whitening

☐ Scaling   ☐ Regular   ☐ Supra   ☐ Deep, with local anaesthetic

Removable Prosthodontics at a Glance, First Edition. James Field and Claire Storey. © 2020 James Field and Claire Storey. Published 2020 by John Wiley & Sons Ltd.
Companion Website: www.wiley.com/go/field/removable

Appendix 2b

Diet (record frequencies per day where possible)

☐ Hot drinks ☐ *Tea/coffee* ☐ *Milk* ☐ *Sugar*

☐ Cold drinks ☐ *Juice* ☐ *Energy/Sports* ☐ *Fizzy*

☐ Sweets/mints ☐ *Sugar* ☐ *Sugar-free*

☐ Snacks ☐ *Fruit* ☐ *Carbohydrate*

Other information:

Positive findings on extra-oral examination: Left(L) Right(R) or Bilateral(B)   No positive findings ☐

☐ TMJ ☐ *Click* ☐ *Pain* ☐ *Lock* ☐ *Crepitus*

☐ Palpable nodes

☐ Muscle pain ☐ *Masseter* ☐ *Temporalis* ☐ *SCM* ☐ *Other* _____

☐ Glands ☐ *Currently suffering from known systemic illness*

Positive findings on intra-oral examination   No positive findings ☐

☐ Palate

☐ Sulci

☐ FOM

☐ Tongue

☐ Lips

☐ Fauces

☐ Gingivae

Relevant information from intra/extra oral examination:

Oral hygiene suboptimal ☐

Initial Tooth, Periodontal and Gingival Examination

Mobility																
TSL (S&K)																
Upper																
	UR8 LR8	7	6	5	4	3	2	1	1	2	3	4	5	6	7	UL8 LL8
Lower																
TSL (S&K)																
Mobility																

Charting Key:

C Crown	**V** Veneer	● Restoration	**PE** Partially erupted
R Retainer	**#** Fracture	○ Cavity	**FS** Fissure sealed
P Pontic	**−** Missing	◉ Recurrent caries	

Basic Periodontal Examination:

Other information:

Appendix 2c

Basic occlusal assessment

ICP	☐ Stable	☐ Unstable	If RCP ≠ ICP, please note CRCP contacts:		

OVD ☐ Normal ☐ Reduced

TSL ☐ Normal ☐ Pathological ☐ Sensitivity present ☐ Dietary and behaviour analysis required

Bruxism ☐ Facets ☐ Ridging/scalloping ☐ Fracture lines

P/- ☐ Acrylic ☐ Co-Cr ☐ Unretentive/unstable ☐ Worn ☐ Unhygienic _____ Age (years)

-/P ☐ Acrylic ☐ Co-Cr ☐ Unretentive/unstable ☐ Worn ☐ Unhygienic _____ Age (years)

☐ Further assessment of prostheses required

Special test and investigations

Radiographic assessment

Please provide a radiographic summary. If necessary, report further in the medical notes __/__/__

Views taken and grade:

Date of last bitewings:

Peri-radicular findings and root canal fillings

Bone levels (%)

Coronal radiolucencies

RF	Root canal filling
PAR	Peri-apical radiolucency
W	Widened periodontal membrane space

UR8	7	6	5	4	3	2	UR1	UL1	2	3	4	5	6	7	UL8
LR8	7	6	5	4	3	2	LR1	LL1	2	3	4	5	6	7	LL8

Bone levels (%)

Peri-radicular findings and root canal fillings

Description of findings:

Results of other special tests:

Further notes:

Appendix 2d

	Diagnoses:	Prognosis	Justification
1			
2			
3			
4			

Risk assessment:

Caries ☐ *High* ☐ *Moderate* ☐ *Low*
E.g. Active symptoms, *poor diet, poor plaque control*, **no history of caries**

Periodontal ☐ *High* ☐ *Moderate* ☐ *Low*
E.g. Deep pockets with bleeding, bone loss, *poor plaque control, smoker, poorly controlled diabetes*, **no history**

TSL ☐ *High* ☐ *Moderate* ☐ *Low*
E.g. >1/3 crown height, symptoms, *<1/3 crown height, poor diet, parafunction, reflux*, **no loss of contour**

Soft tissues ☐ *High* ☐ *Moderate* ☐ *Low*
E.g. Lesion requiring referral, *monitoring lesion, tobacco use, high alcohol intake*, **no lesions**

Endodontic ☐ *High* ☐ *Moderate* ☐ *Low*
E.g. Symptomatic lesion, sclerosed canals, *asymptomatic lesion, simple canals*, **no lesions**

Treatment plan

Prevention and Stabilisation: **OHI +/- gross scale required prior to finalising plan** ☐

See supplementary 6-point pocket chart, plaque score and bleeding ☐

Operative interventions:

Rehabilitation options:

Maintenance plan: *Risks and benefits explained to the patient for each strategy* ☐

Patient involvement discussed ☐

Any other details including recall strategy:

Plan explained to patient ☐
Treatment plan summary provided ☐

Name: _____   Date: _____

Signed: _____

Appendix 3: Referral letters

The Restorative Dentistry Departments in most hospitals will receive hundreds of referral letters each week. Many of these are suitably written, but it is a good idea to ensure that you follow the suggestions below so that your referral letter can be graded appropriately.

It is worth noting that it is considered good practice to grade and sort referral letters using a team approach. This is already happening in some larger centres, where resources allow. Poorly written referrals, or those that do not follow the local protocols or guidelines, will often be returned to you for modifications, or even rejected.

• Ensure that you are using an up-to-date referral template or letter
• Ensure that you have completed all aspects of the template legibly
• Detail the specific reason why you are making a referral, and why the treatment does not fit within primary care dentistry
• Detail if this is for treatment planning, an opinion only, or also for the provision of treatment
• Provide enough supporting information so that the grading consultant can make a decision. Usually this will be:
  ▪ Pictoral charting
  ▪ Basic periodontal examination as a minimum
  ▪ Other relevant indices such as mobility scores, plaque scores, results of special tests
  ▪ Relevant diagnostic radiographs
  ▪ Details of treatment provided to date and the outcome
• For complete or partial dentures, give details of denture design, materials used for construction, and materials used to take impressions
• If patients report problems after provision of treatment, be specific about what they are, and how you have investigated them in the first instance
• Ensure that your patient clearly understand the reason for referral and the time frames involved

Removable Prosthodontics at a Glance, First Edition. James Field and Claire Storey. © 2020 James Field and Claire Storey. Published 2020 by John Wiley & Sons Ltd.
Companion Website: www.wiley.com/go/field/removable

Appendix 4: Partial denture design sheet

Appendix 4 Partial denture design sheet

Partial denture design sheet	
Patient name	
DoB	
Signature of Clinician	
Date	

Design component checklist

Saddle ☐

Rests ☐

Clasps ☐

Indirect retention ☐

Bracing ☐

Reciprocation ☐

Connector design ☐

Maxillary denture design details

Mandibular denture design details

Notes regarding design and discussions with the laboratory

Removable Prosthodontics at a Glance, First Edition. James Field and Claire Storey. © 2020 James Field and Claire Storey. Published 2020 by John Wiley & Sons Ltd.
Companion Website: www.wiley.com/go/field/removable

Recommended and supplementary reading

When compared with other disciplines within Dentistry and wider medical professions, removable prosthodontic techniques suffer from a relatively poor evidence base – this is largely because the majority of clinical stages involve manipulation and application of materials, communication with the patient and the wider team, and the use of specialist equipment; these are very operator-specific skills and as such, the clinician becomes arguably the most critical and uncontrollable confounding factor.

My advice would be to ensure that you are well informed about *possible* prosthodontic tools and techniques – and afford yourself adequate opportunity to test out and play with a range of materials and methods. Settle on materials and techniques that work well in *your* own hands in order to ensure optimal results.

The recommended and supplementary reading below is provided so that you can read around each topic in order to develop your understanding. It is by no means exhaustive. Furthermore, this book is not a reference text – and so it is important for you to engage with and explore the supporting literature further. Many of the classic prosthodontic texts for partial and complete prosthetics are over 50 years old, and very hard to obtain. For this reason, and having reviewed these texts comprehensively, I have mostly chosen journal articles that offer sound practical and clinical advice and are relatively accessible.

General reading	Allen, PF & McCarthy, S (2003) *Complete Dentures – From Planning to Problem Solving*, New Malden: Quintessence.
	Allen, PF (2002) *Teeth for Life for Older Adults*, New Malden: Quintessence.
	Basker, RM, Davenport, JC & Thomason JM (2011) *Prosthetic Treatment of the Edentulous Patient*, 5th edn, Oxford: Wiley-Blackwell.
	Carlsson, GE (2006) Facts and fallacies: an evidence base for complete dentures, *Dental Update* 33(3): 134–142. doi: 10.12968/denu.2006.33.3.134
	Critchlow, SB, Ellis, JS & Field JC (2012) Reducing the risk of failure in complete denture patients, *Dental Update* 39(6): 427–436. doi: 10.12968/denu.2012.39.6.427
	Davenport, JC, Basker, RM, Heath, JR, Ralph, JP & Glantz, PO (2000) *A Clinical Guide to Removable Partial Dentures*, London: British Dental Journal Books.
	Davenport, JC, Basker, RM, Heath, JR, Ralph, JP, Glantz, PO & Hammond P (2000) *A Clinical Guide to Removable Partial Denture Design*, London: British Dental Journal Books.
	Jepson, NJA (2004) *Removable Partial Dentures*, New Malden: Quintessence.
	Lynch, CD (2019) Successful removeable partial dentures, *Dental Update* 39(2): 118. https://www.dental-update.co.uk/articleMatchListArticle.asp?aKey=943
	McCord, JF & Grant, AA (2000) *A Clinical Guide to Complete Denture Prosthetics*, London: British Dental Journal Books.
Accessibility and operator position	Breslin, M & Cook, S (2015) No turning back: posture in dental practice, *BDJ Team* 2: 15164. doi: 10.1038/bdjteam.2015.164.
	Pîrvu, C, Pătraşcu, I, Pîrvu, D & Ionescu, C. (2014) The dentist's operating posture – ergonomic aspects, *Journal of Medicine and Life* 7(2):177–182.

Pre-prosthetic assessment and treatment	Cawood, JI & Howell, RA (1988) A classification of the edentulous jaws, *International Journal of Oral and Maxillofacial Surgery* 17(4): 232–236. doi: 10.1016/s0901-5027(88)80047-x.
	Chapple, ILC & Gilbert, AD (2003) *Understanding Periodontal Diseases: Assessment and Diagnostic Procedures in Practice*, New Malden: Quintessence.
	Devlin, H (2001) Integrating posterior crowns with partial dentures, *British Dental Journal* 191: 120–123. doi: 10.1038/sj.bdj.4801115a.
	Heasman, PA, Preshaw, PM & Robertson, P (2004) *Successful periodontal therapy: a non-surgical approach*, New Malden: Quintessence.
	Ismail, AI, Sohn, W, Tellez, M, Amaya, A, Sen, A, Hasson, H & Pitts, NB (2007) The International Caries Detection and Assessment System (ICDAS): an integrated system for measuring dental caries, *Community Dentistry and Oral Epidemiololgy* 35(3): 170–178. doi: 10.1111/j.1600-0528.2007.00347.x.
	International Caries Classification and Management System (ICCMS).https://www.iccms-web.com/
	McGarry, TJ, Nimmo A, Skiba, JF Ahlstrom, RH, Smith, CR & Koumjian, JH (1999) Classification system for complete edentulism, *Journal of Prosthodontics* 8(1): 27–39. doi: 10.1111/j.1532-849X.1999.tb00005.x.
Impression taking	Besford, JN & Sutton, AF (2018) Aesthetic possibilities in removable prosthodontics. Part 2: start with the face not the teeth when rehearsing lip support and tooth positions, *British Dental Journal* 224: 141–148. doi: 10.1038/sj.bdj.2018.76.
	Field, JC (2016) First impressions count: how to take a primary impression, *Dental Nursing* (12)3. doi: 10.12968/denn.2016.12.2.72.
	McCullagh, A, Sweet, C & Ashley, M (2005) Making a good impression, *Dental Update* 32(3): 169–170. doi: 10.12968/denu.2005.32.3.169.
	Turner, JW, Moazzez, R & Banerjee, A (2012) First impressions count, *Dental Update* 39(7): 455–458. doi: 10.12968/denu.2012.39.7.455.
Managing fibrous ridges and the neutral zone	Allen, PF (2005) Management of the flabby ridge in complete denture construction, *Dental Update* 32(9): 524–526. doi: 10.12968/denu.2005.32.9.524.
	Clarke, P (2016) Managing the unstable mandibular complete denture – tooth placement and the polished surface, *Dental Update* 43(7): 660–662. doi: 10.12968/denu.2016.43.7.660.
	Imran, H (2018) Five steps to flabby ridge success, *British Dental Journal* 225: 597–599. doi: 10.1038/sj.bdj.2018.812
	Lynch, CD & Allen, PF (2006) Management of the flabby ridge: using contemporary materials to solve an old problem, *British Dental Journal* 200: 258–261. doi: 10.1038/sj.bdj.4813306.
	Lynch, CD & Allen, PF (2006) Overcoming the unstable mandibular complete denture: the neutral zone impression technique. *Dental Update* 33(1): 21–26. doi: 10.12968/denu.2006.33.1.21.
Recording the maxillary-mandibular relationship and denture aesthetics	Besford, JS & Sutton, AF (2018) Aesthetic possibilities in removable prosthodontics. Part 3: Photometric tooth selection, tooth setting, try-in, fitting, reviewing and trouble-shooting, *British Dental Journal* 224: 491–506. doi: 10.1038/sj.bdj.2018.222.
	Bishop, M & Johnson, T (2015) Complete dentures: designing occlusal registration blocks to save clinical time and improve accuracy, *Dental Update* 42(3): 275–278. 10.12968/denu.2015.42.3.275.
	McCord, JF & Grant, AA (2000) Registration: Stage III – intermaxillary relations. *British Dental Journal*, 188(11): 601–606. doi: 10.1038/sj.bdj.4800549.
Copying features from existing prostheses	Beddis, HP & Morrow, LE (2013) Technique tips – greenstick modification of dentures prior to the replica technique, *Dental Update* 40(8): 688. doi: 10.12968/denu.2013.40.8.688.
	Jablonski, RY, Patel, J & Morrow, LA (2018) Complete dentures: an update on clinical assessment and management: part 2, *Brtish Dental Journal* 225: 933–939. doi: 10.1038/sj.bdj.2018.1023.
	Soo, S & Cheng AC (2014) Complete denture copy technique – a practical application, *Singapore Dental Journal* 35(12): 65–70. doi: 10.1016/j.sdj.2013.12.001.

(continued)

Designing partial prostheses	Bhola, S, Hellyer, PH & Radford, DR (2018) The importance of communication in the construction of partial dentures, *British Dental Journal* 224: 853–856. doi: 10.1038/sj.bdj.2018.431.
	McCord, J, Grey, NJA, Winstanley, RB & Johnson A (2002) A clinical overview of removable prostheses: 3. Principles for removable partial dentures, *Dental Update* 29(10): 474–481. doi: 10.12968/denu.2002.29.10.474.
	Stilwell, C (2010) Revisiting the principles of partial denture design, *Dental Update* 37(10):682–684. doi: 10.12968/denu.2010.37.10.682
	Walmsley, AD (2003) Acrylic partial dentures, *Dental Update* 30(8): 424–429. doi: 10.12968/denu.2003.30.8.424
Precision attachments: the fixed–removable interface	Thomas, MBM, Williams, G & Addy, LD (2014) Precision attachments in partial removable prosthodontics: an update for the practitioner Part 2, *Dental Update* 41(9): 785.
	Williams, G, Thomas, MBM & Addy, LD (2014) Precision attachments in partial removable prosthodontics: an update for the practitioner Part 1, *Dental Update* 41(8): 725.
RPI system of denture design	Krol, AJ (1973) RPI (REST, Proximal Plate, I Bar) clasp retainer and its modifications, *Dental Clinical of North America* 17(4): 631–649.
	Sayed, M & Jain, S (2019) Comparison between altered cast impression and conventional single-impression techniques for distal extension removable dental prostheses: a systematic review, *International Journal of Prosthodontics* 32(3): 265–271. doi: 10.11607/ijp.6198
	Shifman, A & Ben-Ur, Z (2000) The mandibular first premolar as an abutment for distal-extension removable partial dentures: a modified clasp assembly design, *British Dental Journal* 188: 246–248. doi: 10.1038/sj.bdj.4800443.
Swing-lock prostheses	Alani, A, Maglad, A & Nohl, F (2010) The prosthetic management of gingival aesthetics, *British Dental Journal* 210(2): 63–69. https://www.nature.com/articles/sj.bdj.2011.2
	Lynch, CD & Allen, PF (2004) The swing-lock denture: its use in conventional removable partial denture prosthodontics, *Dental Update* 31(9): 506–508. doi: 10.12968/denu.2004.31.9.506.
Gingival veneers	Alani, A, Maglad, A & Nohl, F (2010) The prosthetic management of gingival aesthetics, *British Dental Journal* 210(2): 63–69. https://www.nature.com/articles/sj.bdj.2011.2
	Hickey, B & Jauhar, S (2009) Gingival veneers, *Dental Update* 36(7): 422–424. doi: 10.12968/denu.2009.36.7.422.
Immediate and training prostheses	Ali, R, Altaie, A & Morrow, L (2015) Prosthetic rehabilitation of the gagging patient using acrylic training plates, *Dental Update* 42(1): 52–58. doi: 10.12968/denu.2015.42.1.52.
	Jogezai, U, Laverty, D & Walmsley AD (2018) Immediate dentures Part 1: assessment and treatment planning, *Dental Update* 45(7): 617.Jogezai, U, Laverty, D & Walmsley AD (2018) Immediate dentures Part 2: denture construction, *Dental Update* 45(8): 720.
Occlusal splints	Adel Moufti, M, Lilico, JT & Wassell, RW (2007) How to make a well-fitting stabilization splint, *Dental Update* 34(7): 398–408. doi: 10.12968/denu.2007.34.7.398.
	Longridge, NN & Milosevic, A (2017) The bilaminar (dual-laminate) protective night guard, *Dental Update* 44(7): 648–654.
	Wassell, RW, Verhees, L, Lawrence, K, Davies, S & Lobbezoo, F (2014) Over-the-counter (OTC) bruxism splints available on the Internet, British Dental Journal 216: E24. doi: 10.1038/sj.bdj.2014.452.
Implants and implant supported overdentures	Laverty, D, Green, D, Marrison, D, Addy, L & Thomas, MBM (2017) Implant retention systems for implant-retained overdentures, *British Dental Journal* 222: 347–359. doi: 10.1038/sj.bdj.2017.215.
	Vere, J, Bhakta, S & Patel, R (2012) Implant-retained overdentures: a review, *Dental Update* 39(5): 370–375. doi: 10.12968/denu.2012.39.5.370.
Principles of restoring maxillary defects	Ali, R, Altaie, A & Nattress, B (2015) Rehabilitation of oncology patients with hard palate defects Part 2: principles of obturator design, *Dental Update* 42(5): 428–434. doi: 10.12968/denu.2015.42.5.428.
	Blair, FM & Hunter, NR (1998) The hollow box maxillary obturator, *British Dental Journal* 184: 484–487. doi: 10.1038/sj.bdj.4809669.

Maintaining adequate oral hygiene	Laing, E, Ashley, P, Gill, D & Naini, F (2008) An update on oral hygiene products and techniques, *Dental Update* 35(4): 270–279. doi: 10.12968/denu.2008.35.4.270.
	Newton JT & Asimakopoulou K. (2015) Managing oral hygiene as a risk factor for periodontal disease: a systematic review of psychological approaches to behaviour change for improved plaque control in periodontal management. *Journal of Clinical Periodontology* 42: S36–46. doi: 10.1111/jcpe.12356.
	Ower, P (2018) Improving uptake of oral hygiene instructions, *Dental Update* 45(9): 893.
Gagging and other difficulties	Ali, R, Altaie, A & Morrow, L (2015) Prosthetic rehabilitation of the gagging patient using acrylic training plates, *Dental Update* 42(1): 52–58. doi: 10.12968/denu.2015.42.1.52.
	Friel, T (2014) The 'anatomically difficult' denture case, *Dental Update* 41(6): 506–512. doi: 10.12968/denu.2014.41.6.506.
	Jablonski, R, Patel, J. & Morrow, L (2018) Complete dentures: an update on clinical assessment and management: part 2. *British Dental Journal* 225: 933–939. doi:10.1038/sj.bdj.2018.1023.
Occlusion and occlusal vertical dimension	Abduo, J & Lyons, K (2012) Clinical considerations for increasing occlusal vertical dimension: a review. *Australian Dental Journal* 57(1), 2–10. doi: 10.1111/j.1834-7819.2011.01640.x.
	Davies, SJ, Gray, RMJ & McCord, JF (2001) Good occlusal practice in removable prosthodontics, *British Dental Journal* 191(9): 491–502. doi: 10.1038/sj.bdj.4801215a.
	Jagger, R (2016) Occlusion and removable prosthodontics. In: *Functional Occlusion in Restorative Dentistry and Prosthodontics*, Maryland Heights: Mosby, pp. 225–233, doi.org/10.1016/B978-0-7234-3809-0.00018-8.
	Wilson, PHR & Banerjee, A (2004) Recording the retruded contact position: a review of clinical techniques, *British Dental Journal* 196(7): 395–402. doi: 10.1038/sj.bdj.4811130.

Index

abutments
    fixed–removable interface, 68–69
    implant-supported overdentures, 83
    retained roots as, 13
    teeth, radiography, 12, 59
access, 15–16
    examination of, 9
    restricted, 17
acclimatisation, 3
acrylic
    gingival veneers, 77
    hygiene, 89
acrylic bases, 37
acrylic dentures, 19
    partial, 56, 57
    surveying for, 65
Adams pliers, clasp adjustment, 71
additions to dentures, 70, 71
adhesives, 27, 29
    immediate prostheses, 79
aesthetics, assessment, 9, 45
alar–tragal plane, 40, 41
alginate, 22, 23, 25
alloy teeth, 70, 71, *see also* cobalt chrome
Alma gauge, 40, 41, 94
altered cast technique, 72–73
angular cheilitis, 9
anterior guidance, 47
anterior repositioning splints, 81
antero-posterior (alar–tragal) plane, 40, 41
Applegate classification, 57
Aramany classification, 84
arc of closure, retruded, 39, 46, 81
articulations
    balanced, 47
    registration blocks, partial dentures, 59
assessment
    aesthetics, 9, 45
    for complete dentures, 8–9
        proforma, 98–99
    for partial dentures, 12–13, 94
    pre-prosthetic, 18–19
    tongue, 21
atrophy, ridges, 15
auxiliary attachments, 69
auxiliary handles, 27

balanced articulations, 47
ball joints, 68, 82
bar joints, 68, 82
bases *see* denture bases
beauty hard wax, 81
bilaminar splints, 81
biological markers, tooth arrangement, 45
blocks *see* registration blocks; wax blocks
bolts, precision attachments, 69
border moulding, 30, 33
bracing, 7, 62–63
bricolage, 3
bruxism, 81

buccal corridors, 41, 94
buccinator, 20, 21, 33
bungs, obturators, 85

c-clasps, 60, 61
candidosis, 9
canine guidance, 47
canine line, 44, *see also* upper smile line
carding wax, 39, 49, 93
cast rests, 71
casts, 36–37, *see also* altered cast technique
    partial denture design, 59
clasp axis, 60, 61
clasps, 57, 60–61, 95
    for casts, 70
    deactivation, 71
    stainless steel, 57
    swing-lock dentures, 74, 75
cleaning, 89
cobalt chrome, *see also* alloy teeth
    cleaning, 89
    partial dentures, 56, 57
communication, 3, 5
    on fibrous ridges, 35
    with laboratory, 15
complete dentures, 95
    assessment for, 8–9
        proforma, 98–99
    immediate, 79
    primary impressions, 22–23
compound materials, 22, 23, 28–29
connectors, 62–63
    swing-lock dentures, 75
contact points, 53, *see also* early contacts; tooth
        contacts
    retruded, 46
    troubleshooting, 91
copy boxes, 54, 55
copying, 54–55, 95
coronoid process, 21
crowns, 61, 65
    milled, 69
    stainless steel, 70
custom trays *see* special trays

dentate trays, 24, 25
denture bases, 36–37, 41
    re-basing, 86–87
denture-bearing area, coverage, 25
depressed ridge form, 8
dexterity of patient
    gingival veneers, 77
    swing-lock dentures, 75
diet, proforma, 101
disto-lingual extensions, 33
dry mouth, 9, 11, 13, 77
dynamic operator position, 16

early contacts, 43, 51, 81, 91
edentulous patient, pre-prosthetic treatment, 19

embrasure spaces, blocking for gingival veneers, 77
examination, 9, 13
    proforma, 101–102
existing prostheses, assessment, 9
expectations, 3
extensions, 6, 7
    assessment, 9
    copying, 54
    denture bases, 37
    disto-lingual, 33
    fibrous ridges *vs*, 35
    peripheral, lower functional impressions, 33
    special trays, 26, 27
    tray extensions, 32, 33
    upper functional impressions, 30, 31
external oblique ridge, 20
extracoronal attachments, 68, 69
extractions, 19
    immediate prostheses after, 79
extraoral assessment, 19

facebows, function, 47
fibrous ridges, 7, 11, 34–35
finished prostheses, 52–53
fitting stage, 53
fitting surfaces, 37, 53
    copying, 55
fixed–removable interface, 68–69, *see also*
        implant-supported overdentures
flabby ridges (fibrous), 7, 11, 34–35
flangeless dentures, 31
flat ridge form, 8
flexible denture bases, 37
fovea palatini, 20, 21
Fox's plane guide, 40, 41, 94
fracture, saddles, 71
frameworks, 70–71
    altered cast technique, 73
    design, 66–67
    maxillary defect restoration, 85
    rest preparation, 61
    try-ins, 70, 71, 95
free-end saddles, 57
    compressive, 73
    impressions, 33
    tray tipping, 25, 73
freeway space, 47
functional analysis, 93
functional impressions
    lower, 32–33
    upper, 30–31
functional sulcus, 21
funnelling, crestal, 12

gagging, 7, 63, 92–93
    training prostheses, 79
    trigger zones, 9, 13
gingival veneers, 76–77
glandular triangle, 20
glass transition temperature, 23, 29

Removable Prosthodontics at a Glance, First Edition. James Field and Claire Storey. © 2020 James Field and Claire Storey. Published 2020 by John Wiley & Sons Ltd.
Companion Website: www.wiley.com/go/field/removable